Psychosocial Well-Being and Mental Health of Individuals in Marital and in Family Relationships in Pre- and Post-Genocide Rwanda

Immaculée Mukashema
Editor

Psychosocial Well-Being and Mental Health of Individuals in Marital and in Family Relationships in Pre- and Post-Genocide Rwanda

palgrave
macmillan

Editor
Immaculée Mukashema
College of Arts and Social Sciences
University of Rwanda
Butare, Rwanda

ISBN 978-3-030-74559-2   ISBN 978-3-030-74560-8   (eBook)
https://doi.org/10.1007/978-3-030-74560-8

Cover credit: Maram_shutterstock.com

This Palgrave Macmillan imprint is published by the registered company Springer Nature Switzerland AG
The registered company address is: Gewerbestrasse 11, 6330 Cham, Switzerland

Contents

Notes on Contributors

Immaculée Mukashema is Associate Professor of Psychology at the University of Rwanda. Dr. Mukashema's research specialties include social pathology, family well-being, marital well-being, marital conflict, mental health, counseling, mapping reconciliation, reconciliation sentiment, and guilt attribution.

Joseph Gumira Hahirwa is Lecturer in Social Sciences & Humanities at the University of Rwanda. Dr. Hahirwa's research focuses on social work, community development, public health, and peace and development.

Alexandre Hakizamungu is Department Head and Social Sciences and Lecturer in Social Work at the University of Rwanda, and a Ph.D. candidate at the University of Gothenburg, Sweden. Mr. Hakizamungu is a licensed social worker specialist with Rwanda Allied Health Professions Council (RAHPC), President of the Rwanda National Organization of Social Workers and a member of the Ethics working group for the Association of School of Social Workers in Africa (ASSWA).

Lambert Havugintwari teaches English, translation and English for Academic Purposes at the University of Rwanda. Mr. Havugintwari's research interests are language teaching methodologies at all levels and assessment of social phenomena in relation to the achievement of SDGs.

List of Tables

1

General Introduction

Immaculée Mukashema

Introduction: Understanding the Concepts Used in the Title of This Book

The term "psychosocial" refers to a concept composed of two words: psychological and social (Long & Cumming, 2013; Upton, 2013). It is known as a shorthand term for the combination of "psychological" and "social" (Stansfeld & Rasul, 2007). Psychological factors include individual-level processes and meanings that influence mental states (Upton, 2013). Psychological factors can be positive, such as happiness, affect, and vitality; or negative, such as anxiety, perceived stress, and depressive symptoms (Long & Cumming, 2013). Social factors include general factors at the level of human society concerned with social structure and social processes that impinge on the individual (Upton, 2013).

I. Mukashema (✉)
College of Arts and Social Sciences, University of Rwanda, Butare, Rwanda

I. Mukashema (ed.), *Psychosocial Well-Being and Mental Health of Individuals in Marital and in Family Relationships in Pre- and Post-Genocide Rwanda*, https://doi.org/10.1007/978-3-030-74560-8_1

1

Psychosocial also implies that the effects of social processes are sometimes mediated through psychological understanding (Stansfeld & Rasul, 2007).

Well-being is a multi-faceted construct described as a state of physical, psychological, and social health. The concepts of happiness, health, positive emotions, welfare, and wellness are considered as the synonyms of well-being (Pressman et al., 2013). A review of the literature suggests that well-being is most comprehensively defined and productively discussed as a combination of the following three components: psychological well-being (PsWB), social well-being (SWB), and physical well-being (PWB) (Pressman et al., 2013).

Psychosocial well-being is a superordinate construct that includes emotional as well as social and collective well-being (Kumar, 2020; Larson, 1996; Martikainen, 2002). Psychosocial well-being is similar to quality of life as they both involve emotional, social, and physical components (Eiroa-Orosa, 2020).

Mental health is "a state of well-being in which the individual realizes his or her own abilities, can cope with the normal stresses of life, can work productively and fruitfully, and is able to make a contribution to his or her community" (WHO, 2004). From the perspectives of positive psychology or of holism, mental health may include an individual's ability to enjoy life and to create a balance between life activities and efforts to achieve psychological resilience (Snyder et al., 2011).

Marriage is a legally and socially sanctioned union, usually between a man and a woman, regulated by laws, rules, customs, beliefs, and attitudes that prescribe the rights and duties of the partners and accords status to their offspring (Britannica & Editors of Encyclopaedia, 2020). Relationships in marriage are vital. They define life context and in turn affect individuals' well-being throughout adulthood (Umberson & Montez, 2010).

Family is understood as a structure reflecting the organization of individuals who are legally bound by marriage and considered of the same relational unit which includes father, mother, and children (Wang, 2013). Relationships in family are essentials to the psychosocial well-being of the members. Family relationships play a crucial role in shaping an individual's well-being across the life course (Merz et al., 2009; Thomas et al., 2017).

Brief Presentation of Rwanda and Its Main Historical Periods

Rwanda is one of the developing countries in the world. It is 26,338 square kilometers in size and is one of the most densely populated countries in Africa. Rwanda's population was estimated at 12,663,116 (NISR, 2020) and it is projected to increase to 16.3 million as a medium scenario of growth by 2032 (NISR, 2014). Among the most known historical referral periods of the history of Rwanda, there is (1) the pre-colonial period situated before 1885, (2) the colonial period starting 1885 and ending 1962, (3) the war of 1990, (4) the genocide against the Tutsis that occurred in 1994, and (5) the post-genocide period.

Pre- and Post-1994's Genocide Against the Tutsis Chosen as the Referral Rwandan Period for the Research Process Presented in This Book

The referral period taken for the outcomes of the field researches presented in this volume is the 1994 genocide against the Tutsis. In this regard, concepts such as "ancient" or "traditional" or "customary" Rwanda which are used in this book refer to the pre-1994 genocide against Tutsis period in Rwanda. The decision of taking the pre-genocide as the referral period to locate the concepts of "ancient" or "traditional" or "customary" is related to the specificities and the conditions under which the research field data were collected.

The selected participants in the research as their full characteristics are presented in Chapter 2 of this book are Rwandan elders with huge experience; and they shared to the research team the perceptions they have about marital and family functioning in ancient Rwanda. However, it was not easy for the research team to be specific on what "ancient Rwanda would mean," especially for the participants in the research. Thus, even if the research team members have obtained the information from the experiences and the perceptions of Rwandan elders with relevant information on marital and family life of the community members in "ancient Rwandan society," the information might have a limitation of the exact period of the history of Rwanda the provided information corresponds to. This could be due to the fact that: (1) the elders might have given information relating to their own marital experience—the youngest was aged 58 and the oldest was aged 98—and simply based on individual perspectives towards the past time of their own lived marital and family life in their own households; or (2) the elders might have given information relating to the experiences they have from what they have observed in marital and family life of their parents; or (3) the elders might have given the information they have heard about marital and family life in ancient Rwandan society.

Consequently, in the analysis of the field data from Rwandan elders as it is described in Chapter 2 titled "A Qualitative Research Approach to Psychosocial Well-Being and Mental Health of Individuals in Marital and in Family Relationships in Pre- and Post-genocide Rwanda," it was not easy to identify the responses linked specifically to the pre- or post-colonial period for instance. The solution to and implication of the above-explained difficulties in situating the historical period of the narrative was that the research team members considered the data to be for Rwandan society in the pre-1994 genocide against the Tutsis period. This is how the pre-1994 genocide against the Tutsis period is named "ancient Rwandan society" in the context of this project. This means that in the later chapters relating to this methodological Chapter 2, i.e., Chapters 3–7, concepts such as "ancient" or "traditional" or "customary Rwanda" refer to the pre-1994 genocide against Tutsis period. Chapters 8 and 9 concern the post-genocide period of Rwanda.

Including both pre- and post-genocide against the Tutsi's periods in the current book is due to the fact that marriage and family life were negatively impacted during the post-conflict period (see, e.g., Bradley, 2018). High rates of domestic violence are seen as a widely observed phenomenon in post-conflict states (Bradley, 2018). Post-conflict in sub-Saharan African societies are associated with intimate partner violence, domestic and family violence (Gupta et al., 2012; Huecker & Smock, 2020; Kelly et al., 2018; Saile et al., 2013).

Research indicates that women and children in post-conflict communities are at greatest risk and are the main victims of domestic violence in post-conflict states (Bradley, 2018; McKay, 1998). Authors such as Aoláin et al. (2011) suggest that after traumatized male combatants leave the battlefield, often their homes become new stages for violence. This is seen as a precipitation of the escalation of violence from the battlefield to the private sphere (Bradley, 2018).

While authors such as MIGEPROF (2011), Mukashema and Sapsford (2013), Ndushabandi et al. (2016), Rutayisire and Richters (2014), Sarabwe et al. (2018), and Umubyeyi et al. (2014) focus on the increase of marital conflict and domestic violence in post-genocide Rwanda, an evidence-based information of reference to the pre-genocide Rwanda period is needed. Thus Chapters 1–7 of this book respond to the lack of academic information on the well-being of married persons and their families in pre-genocide Rwanda.

All the above-mentioned arguments support the reason why we have chosen the pre- and post-genocide periods referred to in this volume. However, it should be noted that the book is not a systematic comparison, but rather a description of the psychosocial well-being and mental health of individuals in marital and family relationships in pre- and post-genocide Rwanda.

Brief History of Mental Health and Psychosocial Support in Rwanda

Mukamana et al. (2019) provide the reader with a general historical and evolving contextual perspective of mental health services in Rwanda, from the traditional healing and mental health services in ancient Rwanda up to the present time. The community members' health in ancient Rwandan society had a perception linked to their beliefs, which would influence the approaches to mental illness. Traditional healing and mental health services in ancient Rwanda considered mental illness as the translation of violation of harmony among the ancestral spirits, with the Almighty God (*Imana*), and with their good relationship with the members of the community (Mukamana et al., 2019). The Western medical practices and mental health services in Rwanda began with the building in 1963, and the official opening in 1972, of a psychiatric hospital at Ndera in Kigali, through the collaboration of a Catholic organization called "Brothers of Charity" with the Government of Rwanda (Mukamana et al., 2019).

In complying with the recommendation of the World Health Organization (WHO) in 1974 about the need for the decentralization of mental health services, a psychiatric dispensary was opened in the southern part of Rwanda and pilot centers were implanted across the country. In those health structures, rural personnel were supported by mobile teams from Ndera hospital (Baro, 1990; Mukamana et al., 2019). Mental health services worked that way in Rwanda until the genocide against the Tutsis in 1994 (Mukamana et al., 2019).

The 1994 genocide against the Tutsis has had serious and challenging impacts on mental health and led to psychosocial problems in the Rwandan population. This challenging situation has been coupled with an important need of proper support: in the aftermath of the genocide, there was a crucial absence of trained professionals in the sector of mental health and psychosocial support to handle these issues caused by the genocide. However, just after the end of the genocide, local organizations and associations were created by Rwandans. These organizations have helped in the trauma healing and psychological assistance (Mukamana et al., 2019). The help provided was given through individual helpful active listening, provided by community-based counselors who were trained while performing the actual helping activities. The support that was given focused quite narrowly on the assistance regarding trauma and psychological problems caused by the genocide and its consequences (Mukamana et al., 2019).

The first national policy of mental health in Rwanda was established only in 1995. Following the establishment of that 1995 mental health policy, academic training of clinical psychologists and social workers started in 1999 at the former National University of Rwanda. The graduates are now supporting in various Rwandan health and psychosocial structures and communities. However, Rwandan professionals specifically specialized in the field of marriage and family therapy are non-existent in Rwanda.

Purpose of the Book

Through the Rwandan oral tradition form of information transmission that was the culture of most pre-colonial societies in the southern Sahara (Smart, 2019; Spear, 1981; Vansina, 1971), Rwandans know that the ancient family used to play a central role in the Rwandan people's life and happiness (MIGEPROF, 2005). If marital and family practices in ancient Rwanda are somewhat known, this has been so thanks to an intergenerational oral framing transmission. According to MIGEPROF (2005), the Rwandan family has trouble keeping up with and adapting to various mutations taking place around it. The assertion can be based on daily observation supported by what is known orally, due to the traditional oral tradition of intergeneration transmission, but written evidence of the past situation on marital and family life in Rwanda is lacking. Such an absence is a big challenge.

Preventing marital and family problems is essential, but preventive means cannot be enough to secure the institutions of marriage and of family against all mental and psychosocial problems which can rise in those institutions. In addition to prevention, therapeutic and psychosocial support strategies for marriage and family health are needed as well. Both prevention and therapy need appropriate policies, which could define practices taking into account the reality of socio-cultural contexts. It is obvious that community members of Rwandan society need a structured marriage and family mental health and well-being preventive strategies and therapy system. Indeed, culture should be a key aspect of all family approaches (Bernal, 2006; Bernal & Sáez-Santiago, 2006).

There is a need for taking into account the uniqueness of the interactions families have with major environmental systems, in applying the Western models to the African and other similar contexts (Jithoo & Bakker, 2011). In his publication on intervention development and cultural adaptation research with diverse families, Bernal (2006) shows the need for research on intervention development and on cultural adaptation of interventions. The same author concludes his article by calling for creative and innovative intervention development research with diverse families to contribute to the body of evidence-based practice with these populations. This volume responds to Bernal's (2006) call.

The book presents an insight into the issues of psychosocial and cultural contexts to be taken into consideration while thinking of creating and implementing marriage and family therapy in Rwandan and in similar societies.

Our book "Psychosocial Well-Being and Mental Health of Individuals in Marital and in Family Relationships in Pre- and Post-Genocide Rwanda" might be the first peer-reviewed book of this kind about Rwanda. The book is meant to be of help to mental health, psychosocial well-being, and the cultural context of marriage and family in community members in pre- and post-genocide Rwanda, and to guide the elaboration of specific policies for mental health and psychosocial support in the area of marriage and family in Rwanda. The book will also help in stressing the importance of culturally evidence-based approaches for mental health and psychosocial support to married and family members in the context of Rwandan society and possibly in similar societies.

Our book is all about the history and nature of marriage and family life in pre- and post- genocide in Rwanda. It falls under qualitative researches. While qualitative approaches are excellent ways to investigate family dynamics and family relationships (Ganong & Coleman, 2014) qualitatively described nature of marriage and family life is rare in the existing scholarship. Qualitative methods allow for getting rich data and exceed quantitative approaches for achieving some research goals (Ganong & Coleman, 2014).

Even during and after the colonization, it is hard if not impossible to find written cultural as well as academic information on marital and family life. One of the most important motives of writing the present book is also to make a milestone in filling the gap, i.e., the absence of academically based information in the area of marital and family life in general and of the well-being of the members living in those institutions of marriage and family in Rwanda in particular.

While available academic publications on marital, family, and family members' lives and well-being in Rwanda are rare, even the few existing ones are focused on the Rwanda post-genocide against the Tutsis. Examples of those researches which are focused on Rwanda's post-genocide against the Tutsis include, but are not limited to: "Intra-family

Conflicts in Rwanda: A Constant Challenge to Sustainable Peace in Rwanda" conducted by Ndushabandi et al. (2016); "Everyday Partner Violence in Rwanda: The Contribution of Community-based Sociotherapy to Peaceful Family Life" by Richters and Sarabwe (2014); A report about intimate partner violence in southern and western Rwanda by Mukashema (2018); "Facing Domestic Violence for Mental Health in Rwanda: Opportunities and Challenges" by Mukashema (2014a); "Psychosocial Factor of Being Street Children in Rwanda" by Kayiranga and Mukashema (2014); "The Challenging Absence of Adults in Youthheaded Households: The Case of Dissension Management Among the Family Members of Households Headed by a Sibling in Rwanda" by Mukashema (2014b).

There are also "Marital Conflicts in Rwanda: Points of View of Rwandan Psycho-socio-medical Professionals" by Mukashema and Sapsford (2013); "Siblings in Households without Parents in Rwanda after the Genocide" by Uwera et al. (2012); "Correlates of Intimate Partner Violence Against Women During a Time of Rapid Social Transition in Rwanda: Analysis of the 2005 and 2010 Demographic and Health Surveys" by Thomson et al. (2015); "Intimate Partner Violence Among Pregnant Women in Rwanda" by Ntaganira et al. (2008); etc. This shows and as was said before, that it is hard to find academic publications about marital and family life and well-being in pre-genocide Rwandan society.

The Book's Approach to Mental Health and Psychosocial Support (MHPSS)

Qualitative data on marriage and family functioning from societies in the pre- and post-conflicts periods where there has been atrocity like that one of genocide in Rwanda, is critical in building a foundation for better mental health and psychosocial support (MHPSS) programming and implementation in health systems. This volume engages with many debates on mental health and psychosocial support in Rwanda, and possibly in other low- and middle-income countries on one hand, and in countries which have faced war and conflict countries on the other hand, or both.

First, there is a question on how to build a foundation for better mental health and psychosocial support (MHPSS) programming and implementation in health systems where there have been atrocity crimes. Second, there is a need regarding how to think about using both evidence-based and culturally informed mental health and psychosocial support (MHPSS) interventions in low- and middle-income countries. Yet, in countries like Rwanda where there has been little extant research on what MHPSS may look like, it is not clear to figure out what evidence-based practice is needed. This is where qualitative research, the inductive research used and presented our book comes in. This book can inform the needed evidence base. That is the most critical massive debate that this book would be contributing to.

Third, the book contributes to understanding what intimate partner violence (IPV) looks like after war/genocide, and what can be done about it. The book also bears out this finding, i.e., that IPV increases in countries where there has been war and conflict, but there is little case illustration of how it looks on the ground, and what is being done about it. Thus, this book would add to that literature too. Fourth, the book contributes to the literature on alternative families such as the raising of children and youth-headed households in societies where there has been conflict and genocide. Fifth, the book contributes to the literature, with awareness of the importance of psychosocial and socio-cultural realities and expectations of the beneficiary communities in order to implement mental health assistance actions without compromising psychosocial and socio-cultural realities.

This volume is aligned with the mandate of the World Health Organization, especially in the Sustainable Development Goal 3 (SDG3) about good health and well-being and aiming at ensuring healthy lives and promoting well-being for all at all ages across all races (United Nations, 2015). Building on the evidence base, it is important to find out how to draw on cultural traditions of communities to solve the psychosocial and mental health problems of the family and its members.

Content of the Book

The book "Psychosocial Well-Being and Mental Health of Individuals in Marital and in Family Relationships in Pre- and Post-Genocide Rwanda" is made up of ten chapters. Chapter 1 is about the Introduction to the book. Chapter 2 is about qualitative research approaches in the book. Chapter 3 consists in the overview of the characteristics of marital life in traditional Rwandan society; Chapter 4 deals with the determinants of marital happiness as a dimension of marital quality in ancient Rwandan society. Chapter 5 is about the socio-cultural causes of marriage destruction in the ancient Rwandan society; Chapter 6 discusses the protective factors of marriage lastingness in the traditional Rwandan society. Chapter 7 describes the prevention and management of destructive marital conflict in pre-genocide Rwandan society; Chapter 8 reports on intimate partner violence post-genocide Rwandan society. Chapter 9 is about children and youth-headed households as alternative family in post-genocide Rwandan society; while Chapter 10 forms the general conclusion to the book.

Conclusion

This book is about the history and nature of marriage in pre- and post-genocide Rwanda. The book sets a milestone toward knowledge of the psychosocial and cultural context of how marital and family life in ancient Rwanda functioned, and with what is now happening in this area in the post-genocide period. The book is based in qualitative research that is rare in the existing scholarship. For societies such as pre- and post-genocide Rwanda, this kind of data is critical in that it would help in building a foundation for better mental health and psychosocial support programming, and its implementation in health systems in societies that have experienced atrocity and crimes such as war and genocide.

While adding a milestone in making evidence-based contributions to the field of marriage and family in Rwanda, and possibly in other low- and middle-income countries, as well as in countries which have faced war and conflict, the book should also be a valuable and useful addition to the field of marriage and family therapy cross-cultural issues, of Africa-focused scholars, and of genocide and atrocity as well as to their consequences on families' researches. The contributors to "Psychosocial Well-Being and Mental Health of Individuals in Marital and in Family Relationships in Pre- and Post-Genocide Rwanda" would like to suggest future researches like this one in other conflict affected states.

References

Aoláin, F. N., Haynes, D. F., & Cahn, N. R. (2011). *On the frontlines: Gender, war, and the post-conflict process.* Oxford University Press.

Baro, F. (1990). Rwanda: Mental care for all. *World Health, 26–27.* https://apps.who.int/iris/handle/10665/52206.

Bernal, G. (2006). Intervention development and cultural adaptation research with diverse families. *Family Process, 45*(2), 143–151. https://doi.org/10.1111/j.1545-5300.2006.00087.x.

Bernal, G., & Sáez-Santiago, E. (2006). Culturally centered psychosocial interventions. *Journal of Community Psychology, 34*(2), 121–132. https://doi.org/10.1002/jcop.20096.

Bradley, S. (2018). Domestic and family violence in post-conflict communities: International human rights law and the state's obligation to protect women and children. *Health and Human Rights, 20*(2), 123–136.

Britannica, T., Editors of Encyclopaedia (2020, March 12). *Marriage.* Encyclopedia Britannica. https://www.britannica.com/topic/marriage.

Eiroa-Orosa, F. J. (2020). Understanding psychosocial wellbeing in the context of complex and multidimensional problems. *International Journal of Environmental Research and Public Health, 17*(16), 5937. https://doi.org/10.3390/ijerph17165937.

Ganong, L., & Coleman, M. (2014). Qualitative research on family relationships. *Journal of Social and Personal Relationships, 31*(4), 451–459. https://doi.org/10.1177/0265407514520828.

Gupta, J., Reed, E., Kelly, J., Stein, D. J., & Williams, D. R. (2012). Men's exposure to human rights violations and relations with perpetration of intimate partner violence in South Africa. *Journal of Epidemiology and Community Health, 66*(6), https://doi.org/10.1136/jech.2010.112300.

Huecker, M. R., & Smock, W. (2020). *Domestic violence* (updated October 15, 2020). In StatPearls [Internet]. Treasure Island (FL): StatPearls Publishing; 2020 January–. Available from: https://www.ncbi.nlm.nih.gov/books/NBK 499891/.

Jithoo, V., & Bakker, T. (2011). Family therapy within the African c. In E. Mpofu (Ed.), *Counseling people of African ancestry* (pp. 142–154). Cambridge University Press. https://doi.org/10.1017/cbo978051197 7350.012.

Kayiranga, G., & Mukashema, I. (2014). Psychosocial factor of being street children in Rwanda. *Procedia - Social and Behavioral Sciences, 140*, 522–527.

Kelly, J. T. D., Colantuoni, E., Robinson, C., & Decker, M. R. (2018). From the battlefield to the bedroom: a multilevel analysis of the links between political conflict and intimate partner violence in Liberia. *BMJ Global Health, 3*(2), https://doi.org/10.1136/bmjgh-2017-000668.

Kumar, C. (2020). Psychosocial well-being of individuals. In W. Leal Filho, A. M. Azul, L. Brandli, P. G. Özuyar, & T. Wall (Eds.), *Quality education. Encyclopedia of the UN sustainable development goals.* Springer. https://doi.org/10.1007/978-3-319-95870-5_45, https://doi.org/10.1016/j.sbspro. 2014.04.464.

Larson, J. S. (1996). The World Health Organization's definition of health: Social versus spiritual health. *Social. Indicator Research, 38*, 181–192.

Long, J., & Cumming, J. (2013). Psychosocial variables. In M. D. Gellman & J. R. Turner (Eds.), *Encyclopedia of behavioral medicine.* Springer. https://doi.org/10.1007/978-1-4419-1005-9_486.

Martikainen, P. (2002). Psychosocial determinants of health in social epidemiology. *International Journal of Epidemiology, 31*, 1091–1093.

McKay, S. (1998). The effects of armed conflict on girls and women. *Peace and Conflict: Journal of Peace Psychology, 4*(4), 381–392. https://doi.org/10. 1207/s15327949pac0404_6.

Merz, E.-M., Consedine, N. S., Schulze, H.-J., & Schuengel, C. (2009). Well-being of adult children and ageing parents: Associations with intergenerational support and relationship quality. *Ageing & Society, 29*, 783–802. https://doi.org/10.1017/s0144686x09008514.

MIGEPROF [Minister in the Prime Minister's Office in Charge of Family Promotion and Gender]. (2005, December). *National policy for family promotion.* Kigali. https://www.ilo.org/dyn/natlex/docs/ELECTR ONIC/92985/117299/F-1037879932/RWA-92985.pdf.

MIGEPROF [Ministry of Gender and Family Promotion]. (2011, July). *National policy on fighting against gender-based violence.* Kigali. Retrieved from https://migeprof.gov.rw/fileadmin/_migrated/content_uploads/GBV_ Policy-2_1_.pdf.

Mukamana, D., Lopez Levers, L., Johns, K., Gishoma, D., Kayiteshonga, Y., & Ait Mohand, A. (2019). A community-based mental health intervention: Promoting mental health services in Rwanda. In S. O. Okpaku (Ed.), *Innovations in global mental health*. Springer. https://doi.org/10.1007/978-3-319-70134-9_36-1.

Mukashema, I. (2014a). Facing domestic violence for mental health in Rwanda: Opportunities and challenges. *Procedia - Social and Behavioral Sciences, 591–* 598. https://doi.org/10.1016/j.sbspro.2014.04.476.

Mukashema, I. (2014b). The challenging absence of adults in youth-headed households: The case of dissension management among the family members of households headed by a sibling in Rwanda. *International Journal of Child, Youth and Family Studies, 5*(2.1), 354–374. https://doi.org/10.18357/ijcyfs. MukashemaI.5212014.

Mukashema, I. (2018). A report about intimate partner violence in southern and western Rwanda. *International Journal of Child, Youth and Family Studies, 9*(3), 68–99. https://doi.org/10.18357/ijcyfs93201818277.

Mukashema, I., & Sapsford, R. (2013). Marital conflicts in Rwanda: points of view of Rwandan psycho-socio-medical professionals. *Procedia - Social and Behavioral Sciences, 82*(2013), 149–168. https://doi.org/10.1016/J.SBS PRO.2013.06.239.

Ndushabandi, E. N., Kagaba, M., & Gasafari, W. (2016). *Intra-family Conflicts in Rwanda: A Constant Challenge to Sustainable Peace in Rwanda*. http://www.irdp.rw/wp-content/uploads/2019/02/intrafamily-con flicts-last-version-2.pdf.

NISR [National Institute of Statistics of Rwanda]. (2014). Size of the resident population 2019. *Fourth Population and Housing Census, Rwanda (RPHC4), 2012, Thematic Report: Population Projections*. http://www.lmis.gov.rw/scr ipts/publication/reports/Fourth%20Rwanda%20Population%20and%20H ousing%20Census_Population_Projections.pdf.

NISR [National Institute of Statistics of Rwanda]. (2020). Size of the resident population 2020. http://www.statistics.gov.rw/publication/size-resident-pop ulation.

Ntaganira, J., Muula, A. S., Masaisa, F., Dusabeyezu, F., Siziya, S., & Rudatsikira, E. (2008). Intimate partner violence among pregnant women in Rwanda. *BMC Women's Health, 8*(17). https://doi.org/10.1186/1472-6874-8-17.

Pressman, S. D., Kraft, T., & Bowlin, S. (2013). Well-being: Physical, psychological, social. In M. D. Gellman & J. R. Turner (Eds.), *Encyclopedia of behavioral medicine*. Springer. https://doi.org/10.1007/978-1-4419-1005-9_75.

Richters, A., & Sarabwe, E. (2014). Everyday partner violence in Rwanda: The contribution of community-based sociotherapy to peaceful family life. *African Safety Promotion Journal: a Journal of Injury and Violence Prevention, 12*(1), 18–34.

Rutayisire, T., Richters A. (2014). Everyday suffering outside prison walls: A legacy of community justice in post-genocide Rwanda. *Social Science & Medicine, 120*, 413–420. https://doi.org/10.1016/j.socscimed.2014.06.009.

Saile, R., Neuner, F., Ertl, V., & Catani, C. (2013). Prevalence and predictors of partner violence against women in the aftermath of war: A survey among couples in northern Uganda. *Social Science & Medicine, 86*, 17–25. https://doi.org/10.1016/j.socscimed.2013.02.046.

Sarabwe, E., Richters, A., & Vysma, M. (2018). Marital conflict in the aftermath of genocide in Rwanda: An explorative study within the context of community based sociotherapy. *Intervention, 16*(1), 14–21. https://doi.org/10.1097/WTF.0000000000000147.

Smart, C. A. (2019). African oral tradition, cultural retentions and the transmission of knowledge in the West Indies. *International Federation of Library Associations and Institutions, 45*(1), 16–25. https://doi.org/10.1177/034003 5218823219.

Snyder, C. R., Lopez, S. J., & Pedrotti, J. T. (2011). *Positive psychology: The scientific and practical explorations of human strengths*. Sage. ISBN: 978-1-4129-8195-8. OCLC 639574840.

Spear, T. (1981). Oral traditions: Whose history? *The Journal of Pacific History, 16*(3), 133–148. https://www.jstor.org/stable/25168470.

Stansfeld, S., & Rasul, F. (2007). Psychosocial factors, depression and illness. In A. Steptoe (Ed.), *Depression and physical illness* (pp. 19–52). Cambridge University Press.

Thomas, P. A., Liu, H., & Umberson, D. (2017). Family relationships and well-being. *Innovation in Aging, 1*(3), igx025. https://doi.org/10.1093/geroni/igx025.

Thomson, D. R., Bah, A. B., Rubanzana, W. G., & Mutesa, L. (2015). Correlates of intimate partner violence against women during a time of rapid social transition in Rwanda: Analysis of the 2005 and 2010 demographic and health surveys. *BMC Women's Health, 15*(1). https://doi.org/10.1186/s12905-015-0257-3.

Umberson, D., & Montez, J. K. (2010). Social relationships and health: A flashpoint for health policy. *Journal of Health and Social Behavior, 51,* S54–S66.

Umubyeyi, A., Mogren I., Ntaganira J., Krantz, G. (2014). Women are considerably more exposed to intimate partner violence than men in Rwanda: Results from a population-based, cross-sectional study. *BMC Women's Health, 14,* 99–110. https://doi.org/10.1186/s12888-014-0315-7.

United Nations. (2015). Resolution adopted by the General Assembly on 25 September 2015. Transforming our world: the 2030 Agenda for Sustainable Development (A/RES/70/1). https://www.un.org/en/development/desa/population/migration/generalassembly/docs/globalcompact/A_RES_70_1_E.pdf.

Upton, J. (2013). Psychosocial factors. In M. D. Gellman, & J. R. Turner (Eds.), *Encyclopedia of behavioral medicine.* Springer. https://doi.org/10.1007/978-1-4419-1005-9_422.

Uwera, K. C., Brackelaire, J., & Munyandamutsa, N. (2012). Siblings in households in Rwanda without parents, after the genocide. *Dialogue, 196*(2), 61–72. https://doi.org/10.3917/dia.196.0061.

Vansina, J. (1971). Once upon a time: Oral traditions as history in Africa. *Daedalus, 100*(2), 442–468. https://www.jstor.org/stable/20024011.

Wang, J. T. (2013). Family, structure. In M. D. Gellman, & J. R. Turner (Eds.), *Encyclopedia of behavioral medicine.* Springer. https://doi.org/10.1007/978-1-4419-1005-9_956.

World Health Organization [WHO]. (2004). *Promoting mental health: Concepts, emerging evidence, practice* (Summary Report). Geneva: World Health Organization.

2

A Qualitative Research Approach to Psychosocial Well-Being and Mental Health of Individuals in Marital and in Family Relationships in Pre- and Post-genocide Rwanda

Immaculée Mukashema, Joseph Gumira Hahirwa, Alexandre Hakizamungu, and Lambert Havugintwari

Introduction

Marriage and family are indisputably important structures for human beings in most societies in the world. The family is a small social unit and a fundamental institution of human society that is formed from marriage. Both marriage and family quality affect health.

Marriage and health are directly related (Robles et al., 2014). Marital functioning is consequential for health (Kiecolt-Glaser & Newton, 2001). Marriage is associated with physical health, psychological well-being, and low mortality (Ross et al., 1990). If marriage seems to be an advantage to married people in terms of mental health (Fincham, 2003; Symoens et al., 2014), marriage should therefore be lived without high or destructive marital conflict. There is the suggestion that destructive marital conflict is a significant risk factor for psychological and physical

I. Mukashema (✉) · J. Gumira Hahirwa · A. Hakizamungu · L. Havugintwari
College of Arts and Social Sciences, University of Rwanda, Butare, Rwanda

I. Mukashema (ed.), *Psychosocial Well-Being and Mental Health of Individuals in Marital and in Family Relationships in Pre- and Post-Genocide Rwanda*, https://doi.org/10.1007/978-3-030-74560-8_2

17

health, and that poor marital quality might lead to overall deterioration in physical health (Choi & Marks, 2008; Segrin & Flora, 2017). Marital conflict has implications for mental, physical, and family health (Fincham, 2003). Marital conflict has been linked to the onset of depressive symptoms, eating disorders, male alcoholism, episodic drinking, binge drinking, and out-of-home drinking (Fincham, 2003).

Marriage protects well-being by providing companionship, emotional support, and economic security. There is a well-established positive association between marriage quality, and physical and psychological well-being (Shapiro & Keyes, 2008). The quality of marital interaction is related to the health of marital partners (Sbarra, 2009; Schmoldt et al., 1989). Marital well-being is an important factor in considering overall quality of life (Larson & Carroll, 2014). The marital relationship is an important factor to married people's mental health. Being happy married is associated with better mental and physical health (Carr & Springer, 2010; Umberson et al., 2013). Marriage may give psychological benefits such as providing enhanced feelings of meaning and purpose, and improving the sense of self (Bierman et al., 2006; Marks, 1996; Reneflot & Mamelund, 2012). Marriage enhances perceptions of well-being for both men and women (Mookherjee, 1997). The quality of marital interaction is related to the health and well-being of spouses (Schmoldt et al., 1989).

Family well-being provides a foundation for positive parenting and child well-being (Newland, 2015). Family relationships play a central role in shaping an individual's well-being (Merz et al., 2009). The quality of family relationships, including social support, can influence well-being through psychosocial, behavioral, and physiological pathways (Thomas et al., 2017).

Contextual Background to Marriage and Family Institutions in Rwanda

In the ancient Rwandan society, the family used to play a central role in the Rwandan people's lives (MIGEPROF, 2005). Social relationships were based much more on the nuclear and extended family, as well as on the neighborhood, than on interpersonal relationships; but those social links in Rwanda have suffered from the tragedies of the last years (MIGE-PROF, 2005). Today's Rwandan society is going through an emergence of nuclear families characterized by individualism, resulting in the disappearance of community life (MIGEPROF, 2005). In addition, Rwanda is facing the problem of destructive marital conflict (MIGEPROF, 2011; Mukashema & Sapsford, 2013).

The importance of destructive marital conflict in post-genocide Rwanda is such that professionals are being consulted by spouses experiencing that problem (Mukashema & Sapsford, 2013). From the MIGE-PROF report (2011), 121 women were murdered by their husbands and ninety-one men were murdered by their wives; twenty-nine women committed suicide because of violence perpetrated against them by their husbands, and forty-nine men committed suicide due to violence they were experiencing from their wives. It is stated that psychological, social, and medical professionals see marital conflict in Rwanda as a growing social and health problem in the post-genocide period (Mukashema & Sapsford, 2013).

Marital conflict, family conflict, and domestic violence have recently gained interest as a new area of scientific research in Rwanda. The interest of research in the area of marital conflict, family conflict, and domestic violence has been influenced by the increase of conflict among spouses, and among parents and children (MIGEPROF, 2011; Mukashema & Sapsford, 2013; Ndushabandi et al., 2016).

The problem of marital conflict has been insufficiently explored in Rwanda (Mukashema & Sapsford, 2013) and only a few researches were conducted in the pre-genocide period in Rwanda. It is noted that most of the few existing number of publications about Rwanda were produced after the genocide against the Tutsis in 1994. That genocide had several consequences including psychosocial consequences and marital conflict in Rwanda can be seen as a legacy of that genocide (Sarabwe et al., 2018).

Among the suggested ways to understand the increase in marital conflict and intimate partner violence in Rwanda are that, it can partially and on the one hand be seen as being among the consequences of the genocide (Rutayisire & Richters, 2014; Sarabwe et al., 2018; Umubyeyi et al., 2014). On the other hand, it can be due to a misinterpretation of gender-related laws by spouses (Ndushabandi et al., 2016), and it can be attributed to the misunderstanding of gender roles and human rights (Mukashema & Sapsford, 2013). Ndushabandi et al. (2016) suggest that legal provisions pertaining to gender equality should avoid contradictions between Rwandan traditional gender practices and Rwanda's cultural values. Also, traditional institutions should not be left out while dealing with family/marital conflict (Ndushabandi et al., 2016). However, it is hard to get a scientific reference on what Rwandan traditional gender practices looked like, or which of Rwanda's cultural and traditional institutions should not be left out while dealing with family/marital conflict.

While concepts such as marital conflict (Mukashema & Sapsford, 2013) and marital discord (Burnet, 2011) are quite newly used in Rwanda (Mukashema, 2014), it is observed that pre-genocide scientific literatures on psychosocial marital and family life in the community members within pre-genocide Rwandan society are rare, if not totally lacking. Research, on the other hand, has slowly started to show the link between the genocide of 1994 in Rwanda and the observed domestic violence in post-genocide Rwanda.

In a research, La Mattina (2017) has examined the long-term impact of civil conflict on domestic violence and intra-household bargaining in Rwanda, and found that women who got married after the 1994 geno-cide significantly experienced increased domestic violence in comparison to those who got married before. Gutierrez and Gallegos (2016) have studied the effect of women's exposure to civil conflict violent events during childhood and early teenage years on the probability that they will experience domestic violence in their marriages as adults. They have found evidence that a potential mechanism through which exposure to the conflict affects domestic violence in the long term is normalization of the use of violence. Rieder and Elbert (2013) have established prevalence rates and predictors of family violence in post-conflict Rwanda. Results from these authors' research indicated that cumulative stress such as exposure to organized violence and family violence in Rwandan descendants poses a risk factor for the development of depressive and anxious symptoms.

We think that in order to be able to fully draw significant conclusions about the variation in domestic violence and to attribute it to conflict and to the post-conflict period, it would be important to have evidence on what the situation of domestic and family violence previously was like. Yet, researches have suggested that the degree of the observed domestic violence in post-genocide Rwanda is linked to the genocide that happened in Rwanda (e.g., Rutayisire & Richters, 2014; Sarabwe et al., 2018; Umubyeyi et al., 2014), or confirm the effect of the genocide on domestic violence (La Mattina, 2017), or attribute the increase of domestic violence to the misunderstanding of gender roles and human rights (Mukashema & Sapsford, 2013), but in our view, some questions need to be answered. They include the following, among others.

The first important research-based evidence needed should be to make sure that all other variables which could play a role in the observed marriage and family instability in post-conflict Rwanda are isolated. Multiple variables such as broader social and contextual determinants of violence including social norms (Linos et al., 2013), honor and shame (Couture-Carron, 2020), religious beliefs (Jankowski et al., 2018) etc., may be linked to the observed extended situation of domestic violence in post-genocide Rwanda.

The second important need is for evidence-based academic information on how marriage and families were doing in terms of functioning and well-being of the members in the pre-genocide Rwanda period. If researchers say that domestic violence has increased in the post-genocide Rwandan period (La Mattina, 2017; MIGEPROF, 2011; Mukashema & Sapsford, 2013; Ndushabandi et al., 2016), and is seen as part of the consequences of the genocide (Rutayisire & Richters, 2014; Sarabwe et al., 2018; Umubyeyi et al., 2014), this would require that the pre-genocide period in terms of marital and family life as well as the well-being of the family members be made known so as to make an academic basis of comparison to the pre- or post-genocide periods. This research would respond to the challenge of this second academic need stated above. It does not intend to establish a comparison between marital and family life in the pre- or post-genocide periods, but instead aims to describe what psychosocial well-being and mental health was like for members in marriage and the family in pre-genocide Rwandan society.

A research project was designed and data were collected from Rwandan elders with perceptions to share on marital and family life in pre-genocide Rwandan society. These Rwandan elders' perceptions on marital and family life in pre-genocide Rwandan society are possibly formed through: (1) personally lived experiences in their own households, (2) observed in their family of origin, (3) or/and or listened to via oral transmission from the surrounding community members. The research team members had ultimately meant to explore, produce, and make available a scientific reference that would describe an overview of psychosocial life, marital and family well-being, marital conflict, and marital conflict prevention and management in the community members within pre-genocide Rwandan society.

The current chapter describes methodological design for a research that intended to achieve the following specific objectives: (1) to identify the characteristics of marital life of the community members within ancient Rwandan society; (2) to demonstrate the conditions of happiness in the family; (3) to evaluate the conditions of the marriage functioning and lasting in the community members within ancient Rwandan society; (4) to outline the factors of marriage destruction; and (5) to describe the ways which were used to prevent and to deal with destructive marital conflict, intimate partner violence, and domestic violence.

Method

Research Design Overview

Research Design

The present methodological design is for both exploratory and descriptive research. It is designed to conduct research in the area of marital processes, characteristics, functioning, psychosocial well-being in marriage and family of the community members within Rwandan society in the pre-genocide period, for which previous scientific references are rare.

Rationale for the Design and Approaches Selected

Qualitative methods standing alone (Levitt et al., 2018) were suitable because they produce rich, detailed, and heavily contextualized descriptions from each source (Levitt et al., 2018). The description of the methodology is detailed as to meet the recommended reporting standards for qualitative research available (see, e.g., Levitt et al., 2018; O'Brien et al., 2014).

Qualitative research approaches allow researcher–participant direct interactions during the qualitative data collection. Direct interactions permit access to subjective and detailed data collection from the participants as one among other advantages of qualitative research approaches as suggested by Rahman (2017). Qualitative methods often lead to extraordinarily rich data and exceed quantitative approaches for achieving some research goals (Ganong & Coleman, 2014).

The focus group discussion was chosen among other approaches for qualitative data collection strategies because interaction between participants in the research using focus group discussions brings out more information than it would if it was done through individual interviews. Compared to individual interviews and surveys, focus group discussion offers an opportunity to explore issues where there is little prior research on the topic (Nyumba et al., 2018). Focus group discussion builds on group dynamics to freely explore the issues in context, in depth, and in detail, without imposing a conceptual framework compared with a structured individual interview (Morgan, 1997; Nyumba et al., 2018). Building on the above reasons among so many others, the focus group discussions were suitable for the current research. Among the five types of focus group discussion (Nyumba et al., 2018), the single focus group which is the interactive discussion of a topic by a collection of all participants and a team of facilitators as one group in one place was used.

Even if the focus group discussion was chosen for its suitability for this research, the research team members were aware of the challenges faced by the approach in data collection. These challenges, among others, included the concern on how the expectations and assumptions of qualitative researchers might influence the research process (Levitt et al., 2018). This awareness led the research team members to continually make self-reflection during the research process.

Study Participants

Researchers' Profile

The principal investigator of the current research holds a doctoral degree in psychology. She is in charge of various courses of psychology related to mental health in the department of social sciences. She is an active academic and has conducted and published several research peer-reviewed articles and book chapters using both quantitative and qualitative approaches. Two research team members are social scientists as well. One of them holds a doctoral degree in peace and development studies. He has jointly conducted several researches using both qualitative and quantitative research approaches and served as a note-taker and moderator during focus group discussions. The other research team member holds a master's degree in social work and human rights. He was also a note-taker and focus group discussions moderator in exploratory research projects. The fourth member is an academic staff member specialized in both the English and Kinyarwanda languages. He belongs to the center of language enhancement of the university that the three other research team members also belong to. This team member also holds a master's degree in development studies. He contributed in tackling the linguistic issues in this research while also bringing in some input as a researcher.

Summary of Participants

A total of forty-five (45 = 100%) elders, Rwandan nationals who had and showed willingness and capacity to provide relevant information on marital life in the community within ancient Rwandan society participated in this research. Twenty-two (22 = 49%) were males and twenty-three (23 = 51%) were females. Participants in one of the focus group discussions were from the "Guardian of memory" known as *Inteko Izirikana* (IN) in Kinyarwanda. This focus group was composed of two males and three females aged between 71 and 78. The "Guardian of memory" is an association of retired elderly people in Rwanda. Its members come together and educate Rwanda's youth about the country's cultural values and norms. The Association is located in Gasabo district of Kigali city. Participants in the second focus group discussion were from Rwanda Elders Advisory Forum (RE). This group comprised five males and two females aged between 59 and 76. The Rwanda Elders Advisory Forum consists of the elderly that are seen as patriotic Rwandan nationals in various domains, including academia, retired civil servants, military and business persons. The forum acts as a "think-tank for national development." The forum is located in Nyarugenge district of Kigali city. All the participants in the two focus group discussions in Kigali city were holders of university degrees (Table 2.1).

The third and fourth focus group discussions, of which one has seven males aged between 58 and 79 and another one that brought together eleven females aged between 60 and 78, were from Nyanza district (Ny), a semi-urban area in the southern province of Rwanda. Participants in these two focus group discussions were of zero years up to six years post-primary education. The fifth and the sixth group discussions, of which one was made of eight males aged between 61 and 98, and the other one with seven females aged between 60 and 90, were conducted in Karongi District (Ka), a rural area in the western province of Rwanda. In this area, the members of the two focus group discussions were of zero up to six years of primary education. The letters put in brackets next to the focus group discussions' full names are different acronyms given to each of the focus group discussions and serve as identifying elements to differentiate them. These acronyms have been used to refer to the concerned focus group discussions in the rest of the text instead of using the full names.

As regards participants' gender homogeneity and heterogeneity, some authors such as Krueger (1994) suggest that generating useful data can be achieved more readily within a homogenous group. Other authors such as Freitas et al. (1998) suggest that mixed gender groups tend to improve the quality of discussions and its outcomes. To satisfy both suggestions

Table 2.1 Summary of participants

FGD characteristics including name, code put in parenthesis, and members by number and by gender	Number of participants	Age range	Level of education	Location
"Guardian of memory" known as *Inteko Izirikana* (IN), mixed: 2 males and 3 females	5	71–78	University degrees	Urban area
Rwanda Elders Advisory Forum (RE); Mixed: 5 males and 2 females	7	59–76	University degrees	Urban area
Nyanza (Ny), 7 males	7	58–79	0–6 Years post-primary education	Semi-urban area
Nyanza (Ny), 11 females	11	60–78	0–6 Years post-primary education	Semi-urban area
Karongi (Ka), 8 males	8	6–98	0–6 Years of primary education.	Rural area
Karongi (Ka), 7 females	7	60–90	0–6 Years of primary education	Rural area
Overall characteristics: (22 = 49%) males and (23 = 51%) females	45	58–98	0 Years of school education to university	Urban, semi-urban and rural area

about gender aspect for the quality of the data in the present research, out of six focus group discussions, two (one in Karongi and one in Nyanza) were composed of males, two (one in Karongi and one in Nyanza) were made up by females, and the two focus group discussions held in Kigali comprised mixed males and females (Kigali city).

Researcher–Participant Relationship

Both the research team members and the participants in the discussions share the same nationality and the same culture, and more importantly the same language, i.e., Kinyarwanda. This was helpful and allowed for good communication free of misinterpretation of ideas shared in the discussion. This could have had some influence on the research in one way or another, but the team members did their best to only stick to their respective roles during the data collection process.

Participants' Recruitment

Recruitment Process

The recommended number of participants in focus group discussions can be six to eight (Krueger & Casey, 2000), four to fifteen participants (Fern, 1982), or ten (Krueger, 1994). The initial plan for the number of participants to take part in each focus group in the current research was to have between six and ten people. However, without the guarantee that all the recruited people would attend the discussion (Levitt et al., 2018), an over-recruitment (Rabiee, 2004) of twelve members was done for each of six planned focus group discussions. Eventually, the smallest focus group had five members present in the discussion while the largest comprised eleven members, which is within the acceptable limits.

Researchers seem to be almost silent on the maximum recommended number of focus group discussions. Glaser and Strauss (1967) suggest that researchers should sample until the point saturation of each category is reached, i.e., when subsequent groups produce only repetitious information. For good results, just a few focus groups are sufficient, as data become saturated and little new information emerges after the first few groups (Carlsen & Glenton, 2011; Morgan, 1996). Most studies use four to six groups because they then reach saturation (Carlsen & Glenton, 2011). For Burrows and Kendall (1997) three or four focus group discussions would be sufficient. Guest et al. (2016) state that almost all themes in a data set can be discoverable within two to three focus groups. In the current research, six focus group discussions were conducted and this number was in the range of the number recommended (e.g., Burrows & Kendall, 1997; Carlsen & Glenton, 2011; Glaser & Strauss, 1967; Guest et al., 2016; Morgan, 1996).

Participants' Selection

Purposive sampling was used since focus group discussion relies on the ability and capacity of participants to provide relevant and deep information (Morgan, 1988). In Kigali city, the recruitment of participants was facilitated by the leaders of the two organizations, i.e., Guardian of memory and Rwanda Elders Advisory Forum that the participants came from. In the southern and western provinces, the recruitment of participants was facilitated by the local leaders at the district, sector, and cell levels. These leaders were initially contacted by telephone and a letter was later on sent to them by email. The content in the email was almost similar to what had been discussed over the telephone. The aim of the email was to officially confirm the number and the characteristics of participants needed for each specified group; and the date and time when the focus group discussions were to be conducted. The local authorities helped in inviting the participants and setting the convenient venue where the focus group discussions were to be held.

The field data preparation and collection was conducted between October and December 2018. No payment was made to participants as compensation for their participation in the focus group discussions. Each participant in focus group discussions held in Karongi and Nyanza districts, however, was reimbursed with the transportation fee they had spent to move from the living place to the administrative place where the focus group discussion was conducted and to go back home. The fee reimbursement could not influence the data because it was provided at the end of the discussion and the participants were not informed about this before.

Data Collection Strategies

Data Collection Procedures

Prior to effective implementation of the research project, the following sequence was observed: (1) the research proposal was submitted to the university of Rwanda for approval and funding; (2) the university directorate of research submitted the research proposal to reviewers who scrutinized it to ensure that scientific and ethical aspects were taken into account prior to approval; (3) the research proposal was presented by the research team in a school seminar to faculty members from various social science schools; (4) a one-day workshop training was organized: the principal investigator facilitated the workshop that served to refresh the research team members on the skills, scientific and ethical behaviors needed for the focus group discussion process. The focus group discussion guide was pretested too; (5) from the university of Rwanda, mission orders were issued to the research team members so that they could travel to the field for data collection.

For each focus group discussion, the research team members and the invited participants would gather in a specific convenient room for a group discussion at each place as detailed under the point: "participants' numbers and socio-demographic/cultural information." The moderator would first welcome all of them. She would all the time work with two research team members, one to serve as the note-taker and the other one to conduct audio recording and collect informed consent forms and transport reimbursement payment form once filled in. The moderator would introduce herself, and so would the two research team members. In turn, each participant was to introduce him/herself as well. Thereafter, the principal investigator would hand a copy of the informed consent form to each participant. This informed consent form contained the following information: words of greeting; introduction of the research team and the institution they were coming from; required age of the participant and the aim and specific objectives of the research; motivation of the research and request of contribution from the participant; rights the participant had to freely participate in the research and to stop contributing at any time during the process; assurance that no name or voice of the participant will appear in the report; telephone number and email of the principal investigator; date; space for signature by a participant (in case of consent to participate). Under the signature on the consent form, the participants were requested to freely provide information on their geographical location and socio-demographic information and they were assured that everything would be kept confidential.

For practical purposes in the context of this specific research, the moderator, with all due respect and ethical consideration, had to seek permission from the participants so that she could first of all read the informed consent form to all of them. That was done and proved to be important for two reasons: (1) the ones who had zero years of education and thus who were not able to read by themselves could understand the content and rationale behind informed consent, (2) all the participants could get the same meaning of the informed consent and some of them would get the opportunity to ask questions for further clarification on the content. After that, the moderator would ask each participant, one by one, to freely choose to be part of the group or not, and would explain that any choice they would make ought not to have any negative consequence.

The above protocol was applied in all the six focus groups. All the participants in the groups agreed to participate and a signed informed consent was obtained from all of them. Following the consent to freely participate in the study, the request would also be made by the moderator to audio record the focus group discussions. During the whole research, all the participants in all groups gave their consent for the focus group discussions to be audio recorded. Prior to the discussion proper, the moderator would state the ground rules to be observed for the good and ethical progression of the discussion.

During the focus group discussions, the facilitator would first of all state each theme, one at a time, in Kinyarwanda, the Rwanda national language. A focus group discussion guide based on the research specific objectives was developed. The statement was formed in an open-ended way. The formulation was for instance: "we would like you to tell us what could be observed as the characteristics of relationship between spouses in the community members within ancient Rwandan society";

one sub-question under this statement was for instance: "what characterized the relationship between spouses in the community members within ancient Rwandan society? We would like you to talk about the strategies which were used to deal with marital conflict in the community members within ancient Rwandan society"; one sub-question for this was for instance: "how was marital conflict dealt with in the community members within ancient Rwandan society? We would like you to tell us about what could be the causes of marriage destruction in community members within ancient Rwandan society"; one sub-question under this statement was for instance: "what were the types of marital conflict that existed in the community members within ancient Rwandan society? What were the causes of marriage destruction, if there was any? What types of marital conflict and domestic violence existed in the community members within ancient Rwandan society?" and so on.

All the stated themes were formulated in relation to the specific objectives of the research. As the discussion was going on, the moderator would restate and reformulate the theme for the participants. In order to deepen ideas, probing open-ended questions such as "can you talk about that more? [following what was said or was given as an added thought by a participant] Can you explain in detail what you mean?" etc.,, were asked by the facilitator as the discussion was going on. The next theme was stated after there were no new ideas coming from the participants. Non-verbal communication and body language expressed by participants were observed and noted as well.

A challenge for the qualitative data collected was the difficulty for the researchers to find out how the Elders participants' perceptions about marriage and family in ancient Rwandan society were formed. Three ways of the formation process of reported perceptions of the participants are possible. The Elders' reported perceptions may have been: (1) a self-reporting on their own lived marital and family experience in their own households; or (2) the experiences from what they have observed in the marital and family life of their parents; or (3) the information they have heard about the marital and family life in ancient Rwandan society. Thus, in Chapters 3–7 the presentation and discussion of the data will be made independently of how the participants' perceptions were formed.

The time spent in each of the six groups was between 60 and 120 minutes as recommended for example by Nyumba et al. (2018). Through debriefing sessions at the end of each focus group discussion, the research team members would indentify some codes for emerging findings from the discussions (McMahon & Winch, 2018). The identified codes were considered during the intensive coding process of the data analysis.

Data Transformation

A one-day training workshop on data transformation was organized. A group of fourth-year students in social work was recruited to get hands-on training in qualitative data transcription. They were specifically trained about the ethical context of the current data. The audio recorded material was transcribed from voices to soft documents in Kinyarwanda. This was done immediately after the data collection. The transcribed data were then translated from Kinyarwanda into English. Notes that had been taken and non-verbal behaviors that had been observed during the discussions were also organized by the researchers and safely kept to support subsequent data analysis and reporting.

Analysis

Considered as a foundational method for qualitative analysis, thematic analysis was applied to identify, analyze, and interpret patterns of meaning within the current qualitative data as suggested by Braun and Clarke (2006). The first step of the analysis was the familiarization with the data by the research team members by reading through the transcribed text, relistening to the voices recorded and writing up initial ideas to be used in the reporting together with the notes taken during the field data collection and debriefing sessions.

The second step was concerned with assigning preliminary codes to the content of each unit of analysis. The unit of analysis was each entire transcript. NVivo software was used to store, organize, and manage the data. Numerous category codes were generated too. A list of quotes was established and the ones used in the report were chosen from there. The third step was all about comparing and compiling codes generated for different transcripts into themes. During the fourth stage, themes were reviewed to complete the analysis and finally, the fifth step was devoted to defining and naming the themes.

Conclusion

This chapter presents the qualitative research approaches used to conduct a research project on the psychosocial well-being and mental health of the members in marriage and family relationships in Rwanda's pre- and post-genocide periods. The overall research significance and implications of the research findings are presented in separate chapters, i.e., in Chapters 3–7. Chapter 3 presents an overview of the characteristics of marital life in community members within ancient Rwandan society; Chapter 4 is about the conditions of healthy marriage and marital happiness; Chapter 5 shows patience and commitment as keys to functional marital life in the ancient Rwandan society; Chapter 6 describes the Elders' views on socio-cultural causes of marriage destruction in the ancient Rwandan society; and finally Chapter 7 is about preventing and dealing with destructive marital conflict in community members within ancient Rwandan society. Each chapter shows the implication of the data presented therein.

The findings from this research are based on perceptions of the participants and therefore may be difficult to generalize. Further extended research and probably with a different approach will be needed. It might be a study comparing marital and family life, as well as the well-being of the spouses and the family members, in the pre- and post-genocide periods in Rwanda.

Acknowledgements This research was conducted through the financial support of the University of Rwanda-Sweden Program.

Declaration of Interest Statement
There is no conflict of interest.

References

Bierman, A., Fazio, E. M., & Milkie, M. A. (2006). A multifaceted approach to the mental health advantage of the married. *Journal of Family Issues, 27,* 554–582. https://doi.org/10.1177/0192513X05284111.

Braun, V., & Clarke, V. (2006). Using thematic analysis in psychology. *Qualitative Research in Psychology, 3,* 77–101. https://doi.org/10.1191/1478088706qp063oa.

Burnet, J. E. (2011). Women have found respect: Gender quotas, symbolic representation, and female empowerment in Rwanda. *Politics & Gender, 7,* 303–334. https://doi.org/10.1017/S1743923X11000250.

Burrows, D., & Kendall, S. (1997). Focus groups: What are they and how can they be used in nursing and health care research? *Social Sciences in Health, 3,* 244–253.

Carlsen, B., & Glenton, C. (2011). What about N? A methodological study of sample-size reporting in focus group studies. *BMC Medical Research Methodology, 11*(26). https://doi.org/10.1186/1471-2288-11-26.

Carr, D., & Springer, K. W. (2010). Advances in families and health research in the 21st century. *Journal of Marriage and Family, 72,* 743–761. https://doi.org/10.1111/j.1741-3737.2010.00728.x.

Choi, H., & Marks, N. F. (2008). Marital conflict, depressive symptoms, and functional impairment. *Journal of Marriage and the Family, 70*(2), 377–390. https://doi.org/10.1111/j.1741-3737.2008.00488.x0.

Couture-Carron, A. (2020). Shame, family honor, and dating abuse: Lessons from an exploratory study of South Asian Muslims. *Violence Against Women, 26*(15–16), 2004–2023. https://doi.org/10.1177/1077801219895115.

Fern, E. F. (1982). The use of focus groups for idea generation: The effects of group size, acquaintanceship and moderation on response quantity and quality. *Journal of Marketing Research, 19,* 1–13. https://doi.org/10.1177/002224378201900101.

Fincham, F. D. (2003). Marital conflict: Correlates, structure and context. *Current Directions in Psychological Science, 12*(23), 23–27. https://doi.org/10.1111/1467-8721.01215.

Freitas, H., Oliveira, M., Jenkins, M., & Popjoy, O. (1998). The focus group, a qualitative research method reviewing the theory, and providing guidelines to its planning. *ISRC Working Paper* (010298), 1–22. http://gianti.ea.ufrgs.br/files/artigos/1998/1998_079_ISRC.pdf.

Ganong, L., & Coleman, M. (2014). Qualitative research on family relationships. *Journal of Social and Personal Relationships, 31*(4), 451–459. https://doi.org/10.1177/0265407514520828.

Glaser, B., & Strauss, A. L. (1967). *The discovery of grounded theory: Strategies for qualitative research.* Aldine.

Guest, G., Namey, E. E., & Mckenna, K. (2016). How many focus groups are enough? Building an evidence base for nonprobability sample sizes. *Field Methods, 29*(1), 3–22. https://doi.org/10.1177/1525822X16639015.

Gutierrez, I. A., & Gallegos, J. V. (2016). *The effect of civil conflict on domestic violence: The case of Peru* (RAND Working Paper Series WR-1168). Available at SSRN: https://ssrn.com/abstract=2851158 or http://dx.doi.org/10.2139/ssrn.2851158.

Jankowski, P. J., Sandage, S. J., Cornell, M. W., Bissonette, C., Johnson, A. J., Crabtree, S. A., et al. (2018). Religious beliefs and domestic violence myths. *Psychology of Religion and Spirituality, 10*(4), 386–397. https://doi.org/10.1037/rel0000154.

Kiecolt-Glaser, J. K., & Newton, T. L. (2001). Marriage and health: His and hers. *Psychological Bulletin, 127*(4), 472–503. https://doi.org/10.1037/0033-2909.127.4.472.

Krueger, R. A. (1994). *Focus groups: A practical guide for applied research.* Sage.

Krueger, R. A., & Casey, M. A. (2000). *Focus groups: A practical guide for applied research* (4th ed.). Sage.

La Mattina, G. (2017). Civil conflict, domestic violence and intra-household bargaining in post-genocide Rwanda. *Journal of Development Economics, 124*(C), 168–198. https://doi.org/10.1016/j.jdeveco.2016.08.001.

Larson, J., & Carroll, S. J. (2014). Marital well-being measures. In A. C. Michalos (Ed.), *Encyclopedia of quality of life and well-being research.* Springer. https://doi.org/10.1007/978-94-007-0753-5_1731.

Levitt, H. M., Bamberg, M., Creswell, J. W., Frost, D. M., Josselson, R., & Suárez-Orozco, C. (2018). Journal article reporting standards for qualitative primary, qualitative meta-analytic, and mixed methods research in psychology: The APA Publications and Communications Board task force report. *American Psychologist, 73*(1), 26–46. https://doi.org/10.1037/amp0000151.

Linos, N., Slopen, N., Subramanian, S. V., Berkman, L., & Kawachi, I. (2013). Influence of community social norms on spousal violence: A population-based multilevel study of Nigerian women. *American Journal of Public Health, 103*(1), 148–155. https://doi.org/10.2105/AJPH.2012.300829.

Marks, N. F. (1996). Flying solo at midlife: Gender, marital status, and psychological well-being. *Journal of Marriage and the Family, 58*(4), 917–932. https://doi.org/10.2307/353980.

McMahon, S. A., & Winch, P. J. (2018). Systematic debriefing after qualitative encounters: an essential analysis step in applied qualitative research. *BMJ Global Health, 3*(5). https://doi.org/10.1136/bmjgh-2018-000837.

Merz, E.-M., Consedine, N. S., Schulze, H.-J., & Schuengel, C. (2009). Well-being of adult children and ageing parents: Associations with intergenerational support and relationship quality. *Ageing & Society, 29*, 783–802. https://doi.org/10.1017/s0144686x09008514.

MIGEPROF [Minister in the Prime Minister's Office in Charge of Family Promotion and Gender]. (2005). *National policy for family promotion.* Kigali. https://www.ilo.org/dyn/natlex/docs/ELECTRONIC/92985/117299/F-1037879932/RWA-92985.pdf.

MIGEPROF [Ministry of Gender and Family Promotion]. (2011, July). *National policy on fighting against gender-based violence.* Kigali. https://migeprof.gov.rw/fileadmin/_migrated/content_uploads/GBV_Policy-2_1_.pdf.

Mookherjee, H. N. (1997). Marital status, gender, and perception of well-being. *The Journal of Social Psychology, 137*(1), 95–105. https://doi.org/10.1080/00224549709595417.

Morgan, D. L. (1988). *Focus group as qualitative research.* Sage.

Morgan, D. L. (1996). Focus groups. *Annual Review of Sociology, 22*, 129–152. https://doi.org/10.1146/annurev.soc.22.1.129.

Morgan, D. L. (1997). *Focus groups as qualitative research.* Sage. https://doi.org/10.4135/9781412984287.

Mukashema, I. (2014). Facing domestic violence for mental health in Rwanda: Opportunities and challenges. *Procedia - Social and Behavioral Sciences,* 591–598.

Mukashema, I., & Sapsford, R. (2013). Marital conflicts in Rwanda: points of view of Rwandan psycho-socio-medical professionals. *Procedia-Social and Behavioral Sciences, 82*(2013), 149–168.

Ndushabandi, E. N., Kagaba, M., & Gasafari, W. (2016). *Intra-family conflicts in Rwanda: A constant challenge to sustainable peace in Rwanda.* http://www.irdp.rw/wp-content/uploads/2019/02/intrafamily-conflicts-last-version-2.pdf.

Newland, L. A. (2015). Family well-being, parenting, and child well-being: Pathways to healthy adjustment. *Clinical Psychologist, 19*, 3–14. https://doi.org/10.1111/cp.12059.

Nyumba, T. O., Wilson, K., Derrick, C. J., & Mukherjee, N. (2018). The use of focus group discussion methodology: Insights from two decades of application in conservation. *Qualitative Methods for Eliciting Judgments for Decision Making.* https://doi.org/10.1111/2041-210X.12860.

O'Brien, B. C., Harris, I. B., Beckman, T. J., Reed, D. A., & Cook, D. A. (2014). Standards for reporting qualitative research: A synthesis of recommendations. *Academic Medicine, 89*(9), 1245–1251. https://doi.org/10.1097/ACM.0000000000000388.

Rabiee, F. (2004). Focus-group interview and data analysis. *Proceedings of Nutrition Society, 63,* 655–660. https://doi.org/10.1079/PNS2004399.

Rahman, M. S. (2017). The advantages and disadvantages of using qualitative and quantitative approaches and methods in language "testing and assessment" research: A literature review. *Journal of Education and Learning, 6*(1), 102–112. https://doi.org/10.5539/jel.v6n1p102.

Reneflot, A., & Mamelund, S.-E. (2012). The association between marital status and psychological well-being in Norway. *European Sociological Review, 28*(3), 355–365. https://doi.org/10.2307/41495128.

Rieder, H., & Elbert, T. (2013). The relationship between organized violence, family violence and mental health: Findings from a community-based survey in Muhanga, Southern Rwanda. *European Journal of Psychotraumatology, 4*(1), 21329. https://doi.org/10.3402/ejpt.v4i0.21329.

Robles, T. F., Slatcher, R. B., Trombello, J. M., & McGinn, M. M. (2014). Marital quality and health: A meta-analytic review. *Psychological Bulletin, 140*(1), 140–187. https://doi.org/10.1037/a0031859.

Ross, C. E., Mirowsky, J., & Goldsteen, K. (1990).The impact of the family on health: The decade in review. *Journal of Marriage and the Family, 52*(4), 1059–1078. https://www.jstor.org/stable/353319.

Rutayisire, T., & Richters, A. (2014). Everyday suffering outside prison walls: A legacy of community justice in post-genocide Rwanda. *Social Science and Medicine, 120,* 413–420. https://doi.org/10.1016/j.socscimed.2014.06.009.

Sarabwe, E., Richters, A., & Vysma, M. (2018). Marital conflict in the aftermath of genocide in Rwanda: An explorative study within the context of community based sociotherapy. *Intervention, 16*(1), 14–21. https://doi.org/10.1097/WTF.0000000000000147.

Sbarra, D. A. (2009). Marriage protects men from clinically meaningful elevations in C-reactive protein: Results from the National Social Life, Health, and Aging Project (NSHAP). *Psychosomatic Medicine, 71,* 828–835. https://doi.org/10.1097/PSY.0b013e3181b4c4f2.

Schmoldt, R. A., Pope, C. R., & Hibbard, J. H. (1989). Marital interaction and the health and well-being of spouses. *Women and Health, 15*(1), 35–56. https://doi.org/10.1300/J013v15n01_04.

Segrin, C., & Flora, J. (2017). Family conflict is detrimental to physical and mental health. In J. A. Samp (Ed.), Communicating interpersonal conflict in close relationships: Contexts, challenges, and opportunities (pp. 207–224). Routledge/Taylor & Francis Group.

Shapiro, A., & Keyes, C. L. M. (2008). Marital status and social well-being: Are the married always better off? *Social Indicators Research, 88*(2), 329–346. https://doi.org/10.1007/s11205-007-9194-3.

Symoens, S., Colman, E., & Bracke, P. (2014). Divorce, conflict, and mental health: how the quality of intimate relationships is linked to post-divorce well-being. *Journal of Applied Social Psychology, 44*, 220–233. https://doi.org/10.1111/jasp.12215.

Thomas, P., Liu, H., & Umberson, D. (2017). Family relationships and well-being. *Innovation in Aging, 1*(3), 1–11. https://doi.org/10.1093/geroni/igx025.

Umberson, D., Thomeer, M. B., & Williams, K. (2013). Family status and mental health: Recent advances and future directions. In C. S. Aneshensel, J. C. Phelan, & A. Bierman (Eds.), *Handbook of the sociology of mental health. Handbooks of sociology and social research* (pp. 405–431). Springer. https://doi.org/10.1007/978-94-007-4276-5_20.

Umubyeyi, A., Mogren, I., Ntaganira, J., & Krantz, G. (2014). Women are considerably more exposed to intimate partner violence than men in Rwanda: Results from a population-based, cross-sectional study. *BMC Women's Health, 14*, 99–110. https://doi.org/10.1186/s12888-014-0315-7.

3

An Overview of the Characteristics of Marital Life in Traditional Rwandan Society

Immaculée Mukashema, Joseph Gumira Hahirwa, Alexandre Hakizamungu, and Lambert Havugintwari

Introduction

One of the central functions of marriage is to create a family and to define relationships between the spouses in the family. It is suggested that family organization is a central aspect of cultural identity (McDonald, 2000). The timing of changes in family life can vary depending on the society and culture (Hewitt & Churchill, 2020). Countries across the world have put in place policies related to marriage and family, but it may be difficult to implement and to enforce those policies, due to the strength of traditional family and marriage practices (Hewitt & Churchill, 2020; Kim et al., 2013; Koski et al., 2017; Maswikwa et al., 2015).

This chapter presents the outcomes from a research about the characteristics of marital and family life in ancient Rwandan society. The

I. Mukashema (✉) · J. Gumira Hahirwa · A. Hakizamungu · L. Havugintwari
College of Arts and Social Sciences, University of Rwanda, Butare, Rwanda

© The Author(s), under exclusive license to Springer Nature Switzerland AG 2021
I. Mukashema (ed.), *Psychosocial Well-Being and Mental Health of Individuals in Marital and in Family Relationships in Pre- and Post-Genocide Rwanda*, https://doi.org/10.1007/978-3-030-74560-8_3

research field data were collected during focus group discussions with Rwandan elders. The focus group discussions brought together a mixed group made up of two males and three females selected in the "Guardian of memory" known as *Inteko Izirikana* (IN) located in Kigali city; a mixed group made up of five males and two females from Rwanda Elders Advisory Forum (RE) in Kigali City; two homogeneous groups made up of seven males and eleven females respectively selected in the district of Nyanza (Ny) of the southern province of Rwanda; and two homogeneous groups made up of eight males and seven females respectively selected in the district of Karongi (Ka) of the western province of Rwanda.

The data were collected and analyzed using methodological approaches as detailed in Chapter 2 of this volume.

Characteristics of Marital and Family Life in Customary Rwanda

Marital life in customary Rwandan society had a number of characteristics. The marital life was characterized by compliance with values within the household. There were spousal specific responsibilities in the household and special gender complementarities. The bearing and the upbringing of children was done in the cultural setting of gender roles in ancient Rwandan society. The parents' mindset toward their children was all about preparing them to become future good spouses. In the community within pre-genocide Rwandan society, the marriage was a project in which the family had an important role to play. Prior to the marriage day, the young people would receive verbal advice to guide them on how marital and family life should be conducted.

Marital Life Characterized by Compliance with Values Within the Household

In the customary Rwandan society, marital life was guided by compliance with a number of cultural and behavioral values. The values that were observed include mutual respect, mutual love, spousal harmony, faithfulness, and unity among the household members. The spouses had a responsibility to practice and show good behaviors so as to serve as "role models" to the children in daily marital life in the households.

> Spouses in the customary Rwandan society had to show good behaviors based on mutual respect and love so that their children could grow up in that same perspective of behaving well. That life framework would give a good example of marital life to the children. (Ka, male)

> Husband and wife were living harmoniously and respected each other. The husband respected his wife and the wife respected her husband. The same could even be observed between themselves and their children. As a result, they could all get on very well with each other at home. (Ny, male)

Family values are beliefs about what is right, wrong, or important in life that people often learn through socialization from their families, typically being the importance of high moral standards and the traditional family unit of mother, father, and children (Oxford Learner's Dictionaries, 1948). According to the Rwandan elders, the respect between the spouses rested on the principle that the husband was considered as the respected chief of the household. After the fulfillment of his home's responsibilities such as land labor, the husband used to go out, meet his fellow men and socialize with them. When back home, the wife would show her husband the respect he deserved as the chief of the household.

> The husband as chief of the household was respected. For instance, after working in the farm, or fulfilling other household obligations, he would go to gather with his fellow men in the open talk. When he was later on back home, the wife would welcome him and show respect to him as chief of the household. (Ny, male)

> The husband was aware of the fact that he was a man and the wife was aware that she was a woman, they had to respect each other. (Ny, male)

There is a fact that in some African societies women were socialized to be self-effacing and that was not seen as an oppression exercised by men to women (Hinga et al., 2008). But in the views of Rwandan elders who participated in this study, the respectful consideration of the husband as chief of the household by the wife was culturally done under the mutual respect and love among other values, and this would tremendously lead to harmony in the household. The spouses, men and women, who respected the Rwandan culture, had to observe cultural values that required them to show mutual respect. Thus, the woman could give good advice to her husband and the latter would normally not object, and vice versa, in order to have a good functional household. The wives were the close collaborators of their husbands in terms of decision-making in the households.

Each spouse had her/his own responsibilities to be accomplished with respect within the household life, the wives would be the managers of the household. (RE, male)

The wife was so respected that no husband could offer a cow to someone without discussing this with his wife or without her consent. (IN, male)

Spousal Specific Responsibilities in the Household and Gender Complementarities

In the ancient Rwandan society, the spouses were aware of the constitutional/biological differences between them. As chief of the household, the husband was there to acknowledge that he was a "man" and thus was supposed to assume his responsibilities consequently. In terms of spouses' relationship, the husband's responsibilities consisted among so many others in giving his wife a significant value. On her side, the wife had to recognize that she was a "woman" and should recognize that her husband was the chief of the household; and thus deserved unconditional respect. Each of the spouses had a specific way of maintaining the spousal relationship at home. This depended on what the man would expect from his wife and what his wife would expect from him. They had to please and complement each other.

> The spouses' life in the ancient households of Rwandan society was that each spouse had his or her specific responsibilities. The wife was culturally given the duties of ensuring domestic cleanliness and properly keeping the milk jars, dishes, and bed. All those were the duties of the wife. Building a hut (traditional Rwandan living shelter) was the responsibility of the husband. He also had to repair it whenever necessary. (IN, male)

> The wife and the husband had a responsibility of complementing each other. The wife was in charge of the house ground, she was engaged in the good managementwife was in charge of the house ground, she was engaged in the good management of the household's resources too. She had to care for the kids and the guests and to carry out any other domestic activity. (IN, female)

> The husband and the wife used to be complementary. The complementarities were not only limited to procreation. The wife had some other responsibilities like caring for grains, food, and feeding children, while the husband was in charge of searching for the household's wealth. The spouses used to have gender-based specificities but also gender complementarities because the wife had to please her husband and vice versa. (RE, male)

The Rwandan elders who participated in the focus group discussion said that the spouses in the ancient Rwandan society respected and valued their biological differences and complemented each other. Each spouse had, knew, and would never complain about his or her specific responsibilities in the household. The wife would stay at home as care giver in the household while the husband was in charge of searching and increasing the household's wealth, like in some other traditional African societies (Kanji & Schober, 2013).The responsibilities of the spouses in the households in ancient Rwandan society were based on gender difference and on complementarities. The views of the elders who participated in this study about men/women relationships in the context of the ancient Rwandan society are far from the literature stressing that the African women have been culturally seen as having always been oppressed, discriminated against because of the notion that they would only become wives and mothers (Adekunle, 2007; Rosaldo & Lamphere, 1974). In the ancient Rwandan society, the normal Rwandan marital and family relationship particularly, was characterized by the cultural context of husband/wife relationships of living in complementarities based on gender differences. This did not necessarily mean oppression and discrimination; according to the Rwandans elders. Instead, this contributed to marital and family well-being leading to family stability, which benefited the family members in ancient Rwandan society. This is consistent with the fact that relationships with family members are significant for well-being across the life course (Merz et al., 2009; Umberson et al., 2010), and subjective well-being and relationship quality contribute to the health benefits of marriage (Lawrence et al., 2019).

Bearing and Upbringing of Children with Respect to Gender Roles

In ancient Rwandan society, the two spouses had to produce children and make the family larger and extended. The parents would raise their children and ensure they got an appropriate upbringing in accordance with the Rwandan "cultural" context. Everything was done to ensure that specific gender and gender role difference were respected.

> The spouses would procreate and expand the family. Their children would grow up having a bit of the culture from their parents. The children would follow the lifestyle that was displayed to them by their parents. (Ka, male)

> The parents had to take care of their children and give them a good upbringing. The children would grow up and show their family culture. At the time of customary Rwandan society, children could not be seen wandering in the street as it happens today. (Ny, male)

The current findings about the characteristics of marital and family life in ancient Rwandan society meet the family culture or family tradition understanding as an aggregate of attitudes, ideas and ideals, and environment, which a person inherits from his/her parents and ancestors (Wikipedia Encyclopedia, 2001). The findings show that the children used to follow the life model of their parents in order to acquire the social behavior in the cultural context of the Rwandan society. The parents had to take care of their children and do their best so that the behavior of the latter could not conflict with the Rwandan cultural context. In this logic, it was impossible to find children growing up in the streets in the ancient Rwandan society.

Even if this study's objective is not a comparison between family life in ancient and contemporary Rwandan society, but an exploration and description of the characteristics of marital life in customary Rwandan society, it is stated that the 1994 genocide against the Tutsis has had a number of negative consequences: the decline of ancient family structure and functioning; and the economic and psychosocial consequences as well as the increasing marital conflict, which have had a particular influence on the new phenomenon of street children in Rwanda (Kayiranga & Mukashema, 2014). The 1994 genocide has been a "fertile land" for the real, serious, and constantly increasing phenomenon of street children (MIGEPROF, 2005).

Parents' Mindset with Regard to Preparing Their Children to Become Future Good Spouses

In their daily lifestyles and activities, the parents always felt concerned about, and minded the preparation of their children for marriage in the future. The way the parents lived in their daily life would prepare their children to become future spouses and parents. Through the parents' family life dynamic in the home, the children would learn how a wife and how a husband had to behave within the household. The children, in watching the behaviors of their parents in their daily life, could figure out how to behave as spouses and as parents. Both parents had to get rid of indecent behaviors in the eyes of their children. They were careful in their behaviors especially in front of their children. They would strive to avoid that their children see or find anything wrong in them. The parents had various activities to perform that were to be learned by the children. Particularly from the mother, a young girl was practically prepared about the details of caring for a home, and also on how to behave in case of any problems with her husband. On the other hand, the young boy would mainly learn from his father's behavior.

> When raised in their family, the girl and the boy used to observe and learn from their parents' behaviors. The young lady used to especially observe her mother. She was learning to prepare milk. This is the culture that his mother would give her. She was shown how to cook food. The mothers would teach their daughters how to make a bed and do cleanliness. The young boys would particularly observe their fathers' behaviors. They used to observe how the parents were living together and how a man would have to behave when living with his wife once married. (Ny, female)

> A girl would only start new life in her own household when she was ready to behave as a wife. Her marriage only could take place after she had done all practical exercises in the family, after she had come to know how to make a bed, sweep, prepare milk, and handle all household chores. (IN, female)

> A young lady was raised by her mother and trained about appropriate behaviors required to sustain her new family/household and how she would need to behave. The mother would also teach her how to be seen as exemplary among other girls. The mother could not allow her daughter to go outside of the house ground. She would protect her from contact with males to preserve her virginity until she got married. (IN, male)

> The parents had to do all their best so that their children could not see or hear something wrong from them. For example, the parents had to avoid mistakes such as severely and heavily blaming the partner in the eyes of their children or having bad discussions in the presence of the children. (Ny, female)

While the children would learn from both parents in general, the young lady was always focused on learning from her mother, while the young boy would do the same from his father. The girls would learn to become good wives and the boys had to do alike to become good husbands. The boys would be trained specifically in how a man had to behave to be seen as a chief of the household and how to live with a wife. The parents would try to protect their children so that they could stay with their virginity until they get married. That was so important especially for the girl. In traditional African societies, virginity was held in high esteem. The parents of a married virgin bride would receive special tribute from the groom's family for a successful upbringing of their daughter. This tribute conferred to the bride unique respect from her in-laws (Chereji & King, 2015).

The Marriage Project in the Ancient Rwandan Society and the Important Role of the Family

In the ancient Rwandan society, marriage was a project that required some preparations. When it was high time for a young boy to get married, his father was in charge of making a home for a prospective household. In general, no boy was to be aged twenty-five or above before his parents had helped or pushed him to get married. The move would come two ways. Either of the parents would judge that their son was ready to get married or the young boy himself could express his wish to the parents that he wanted to have a wife. Once this was agreed upon, the parents of the young boy were responsible for the initiation of their son's marriage process. This process of marriage would normally start in the son's family which had to look for a bride who was suitable for the boy. While looking for a good bride for the son, the father often had to do everything through another person known as a "marriage mediator." The marriage mediator was a man or a woman, socially well known in the community and close to the son's family. His/her role was to look for a prospective bride for the boy ready to be a groom. The marriage mediator was meant to initiate the discussion with the parents in the family of a girl so as to get their agreement and eventually propose her as a future bride to the young man.

In order to get married in the ancient Rwandan society, the boy's father had the responsibility to evaluate and judge if it was time for him to make a home for his son. However, the boy himself as well could tell his parents that he wanted to have his own home. (IN, male)

The son's father was the one in charge of making a home for his son and searching for the prospective bride. The practice was that the father had to get a great friend of his to be the "marriage mediator" and ask him/her to look for a young lady who would fit and suit his son as a wife. The marriage mediator would first search for a family with good reputation and in which there was a young girl, with good behaviors. Then, he/she went to tell the parents of the girl: ["Somebody has asked me to search for a beautiful and humble bride, who has got good upbringing from her parents. The reason why I have come to you is that I know your good habits and the way you live within your home. It seems your daughter looks mature now. I am wondering if you can let her get married if ever if I introduce a good man to her? Would you be willing to give her to him?"]. (Ny, female)

In ancient Rwandan society, of course only the groom and the bride would get together to make a household but this was simply the result of collaboration between their two families of origin. The families would collaborate and make all the arrangements to marry their two young people. The bride was to become a wife because she had to work as a kind of "bridge" linking two families [her own family and the one of her husband]. (IN, female)

The marriage of two young people was a way of strengthening their two families of origin. For the two families to have their two young children get married, there was a condition. Everything depended on the way each of the two families was socially appreciated in terms of the upbringing given to the children and the way the family members were appreciated in terms of behaviors. (RE, female)

In the customary Rwandan society and in some other African societies, for the young people to get married, they would not decide or choose their partners by themselves (Ndoromo & Banyanga, 2019). The parents and the families' members would play a crucial role in assisting their daughter or son in selecting a marital partner (Adekunle, 2007). In the traditional Rwandan society like in some other African societies, the marriage was seen as a union beyond the two individuals and thus as a permanent union between a man and his wife, as well as of their two respective families (Arugu, 2014). The two respective families of the groom and the bride would play a major role in initiating initiation and preparation of the marriage. The marriage was a way of strengthening two families. To be chosen as a family in-law in African traditional societies, the family background was investigated. The family was not to be characterized by any of the following problems: absence of virginity, existence of insanity, violent behaviors, incurable or contagious diseases, immorality, divorce, and stealing (Chereji & King, 2015).

Verbal Advice to the Young People Prior to Their Marriage Day

When the time for marriage time was getting near, close relatives as well as the parents of the bride and groom used to provide each of the prospective spouses with some verbal advice so as to bring to their attention that marriage is a life that needs to be taken great care of. Some of such pieces of advice would be the provision of verbal instructions which could help the new spouses to cope with challenges in their daily marital life. The young people about to get married would also get some advice about the consideration they ought to have toward their families-in-law. It was made clear that the latter would be their new parents in whom to place their trust. Additionally, they would be reminded of the responsibilities they had to assume. This included avoiding any behavior that could disrupt the reputation of their families of origin in the families-in-law. The gender aspects were considered while giving advice, i.e., the uncles would give advice to the groom while the aunts would do the same to the bride.

Just prior getting married, the girl's aunts would give her instructions on the way she should behave and on how to cope with problems that may occur in her new home. The young man's uncles also used to advise the young man on how to build and sustain the home. (RE, female)

The parents used to advise both the groom and the bride as follows: ["Listen to me my son, you are going to marry, leave behind your vices and bad behaviors. If you used to behave this or that way, for example coming back to our home late in the evenings, beware and know very well that this will no longer be the case"]. They would also tell the girl: ["The most important thing among others is taking care of your husband. Please take care of him properly"]. (Ny, female)

When the young girl or the young boy was about to get married, the advice to her or to him from the parents was like: ["Please our child, take care of your spouse, and do not behave in a way that could disrupt our reputation"]. This really was helping and putting the new spouses in a situation of awareness whereby they had to resolve any issue or misunderstanding between them as quickly and as discreetly as possible so that it could not be known by other people, i.e., the public. (RE, male)

Giving advice to the young people before/prior to the marriage ceremony was common among other African customary societies. (Amos, 2013)

Conclusion

Normal spousal life in customary Rwandan society was characterized by observing cultural and behavioral values in a household. There were close collaboration and complementarities between the spouses. The spouses were taught to see each other as equal partners, and this was observed through mutual respect that characterized them, despite the fact of the differences in their biological constitutions in certain aspects making them "male" and "female." Their constitutional difference was, however, an asset that allowed favorable complementarities of spouses in their households because of some specific gender responsibilities. The children were growing up in a household and such a place was considered to be a learning environment to acquire good behaviors. The daily lifestyle of the spouses in ancient Rwandan society was a way of preparing their children for their own marriage in the future. The parents would play a huge role in the marriage of their children. The perceptions of the participants about the characteristics of marital life in traditional Rwandan society did not show divergent position based on the gender or on the geographical location of the Rwandan elders participants in the research.

The findings from the field research presented in this chapter will be of interest to, but not only limited to, the following people: the participants in the current study, young people about to get married, policymakers, religious authorities, and married people. Even if data from focus group discussions may not be generalized, the cultural context of the current findings allow for an insight into what marital life in the ancient Rwandan society was like. It is true that some experiences can be taken from those earlier times, get built on and adapted for home-grown solutions for healthier marital lifestyles in today's Rwandan society.

Acknowledgements This research was conducted through the financial support of the University of Rwanda-Sweden Program.

Declaration of Interest Statement
There is no conflict of interest.

References

Adekunle, J. O. (2007). *Culture and customs of Rwanda*. Greenwood Press.

Amos, P. M. (2013, December 18). *Parenting and culture: Evidence from Some African Communities*. https://www.intechopen.com/books/parenting-in-south-american-and-african-contexts/parenting-and-culture-evidence-from-some-african-communities.

Arugu, L. O. (2014). Social indicators and effects of marriage divorce in African societies. *The Business & Management Review, 4*(4), 374–383.

Chereji, C.-R., & King, C. W. (2015). Aspects of traditional conflict management practices among the Ogoni of Nigeria. *Conflict Studies Quarterly, 10*, 56–68.

Hewitt, B., & Churchill, B. (2020). Convergence and difference: Marriage and family life from a cross-cultural perspective. In W. Kim Halford & F. Van De Vijver (Eds.), *Cross-cultural family research and practice* (pp. 57–102). https://doi.org/10.1016/B978-0-12-815493-9.00003-X.

Hinga, T. M., Kubai, A. N., Mwaura, P., & Ayanga, H. (2008). *Women, religion and HIV/AIDS in Africa: Responding to ethical and theological challenges.* Cluster Publications.

Kanji, S., & Schober, P. (2013). Are couples with young children more likely to split up when the mother is the main or an equal earner?. *Journal of Sociology, 48*(74), 38–58. https://doi.org/10.1177/0038038512467710.

Kayiranga, G., & Mukashema, I. (2014). Psychosocial factor of being street children in Rwanda. *Procedia-Social and Behavioral Sciences, 140*, 522–527. https://doi.org/10.1016/j.sbspro.2014.04.464.

Kim, M., Longhofer, W., Boyle, E. H., & Nyseth, H. (2013). When do laws matter? National minimum-age-of-marriage laws, child rights, and adolescent fertility, 1989–2007. *Law & Society Review, 47*(3), 589–619. https://doi.org/10.1111/lasr.12033.

Koski, A., Clark, S., & Nandi, A. (2017). Has child marriage declined in sub-Saharan Africa? An analysis of trends in 31 countries. *Population and Development Review, 43*(1), 7–29. https://doi.org/10.1111/padr.12035.

Lawrence, E. M., Rogers, R. G., Zajacova, A., & Wadsworth, T. (2019). Marital happiness, marital status, health, and longevity. *Journal of Happiness Studies, 20*, 1539–1561. https://doi.org/10.1007/s10902-018-0009-9.

Maswikwa, B., Richter, L., Kaufman, J., & Nandi, A. (2015). Minimum marriage age laws and the prevalence of child marriage and adolescent birth: Evidence from Sub-Saharan Africa. *International Perspectives on Sexual and Reproductive Health, 41*(2), 58–68. https://doi.org/10.1363/4105815.

McDonald, P. (2000). Gender equity in theories of fertility transition. *Population and Development Review, 26*(3), 427–439. https://doi.org/10.1111/j.1728-4457.2000.00427.x.

Merz, E.-M., Consedine, N. S., Schulze, H.-J., & Schuengel, C. (2009). Well-being of adult children and ageing parents: Associations with intergenerational support and relationship quality. *Ageing & Society, 29*, 783–802. https://doi.org/10.1017/s0144686x09008514.

MIGEPROF [Minister in the Prime Minister's Office in Charge of Family Promotion and Gender]. (2005, December). *National policy for family promotion.* Kigali. https://www.ilo.org/dyn/natlex/docs/ELECTRONIC/92985/117299/F-1037879932/RWA-92985.pdf.

Ndoromo, O., & Banyanga, J. A. (2019). Cultural impact and an intimate partner aggression in African societies: A comparison of Rwanda and South Sudan. *European Journal of Social Sciences, 1*(3). 170–177. http://dx.doi.org/10.26417/ejss.v1i3.p170=177.

Oxford Learner's Dictionaries. (1948). *Family values.* https://www.oxfordlearnersdictionaries.com/definition/english/family-values.

Rosaldo, M. Z., & Lamphere, L. (1974). *Women, culture & society.* Stanford University Press.

Umberson, D., Pudrovska, T., & Reczek, C. (2010). Parenthood, childlessness, and well-being: A life course perspective. *Journal of Marriage and Family, 72*(3), 612–629. https://doi.org/10.1111/j.1741-3737.2010.00721.x.

Wikipedia Encyclopedia. (2001). *Family traditions.* https://en.wikipedia.org/wiki/Family_traditions.

4

Determinants of Marital Happiness as a Dimension of Marital Quality in Ancient Rwandan Society

Immaculée Mukashema, Joseph Gumira Hahirwa, Alexandre Hakizamungu, and Lambert Havugintwari

Introduction

Life happiness was conceptualized as a positive emotional state that persists over extended periods, irrespective of temporary fluctuations in affect level (Argyle, 1999). Spanier and Lewis (1980) suggest that the quality of marital relationships and concepts such as happiness, satisfaction, adjustment continue to be the most widely studied in the field. Happiness might be good for both the mind and the body (Kushlev et al., 2020). Happiness may be understood as concerning what benefits an individual, makes him/her feel better, serves his/her interests and goals and, ultimately, is good and desirable for him/her (Lavazza, 2016). Happiness is the ultimate form of pleasure without which all other things are considered to be incomplete (Patel & Dhar, 2018).

I. Mukashema (✉) · J. Gumira Hahirwa · A. Hakizamungu ·
L. Havugintwari
College of Arts and Social Sciences, University of Rwanda, Butare, Rwanda

© The Author(s), under exclusive license to Springer Nature
Switzerland AG 2021
I. Mukashema (ed.), *Psychosocial Well-Being and Mental Health of Individuals in Marital and in Family Relationships in Pre- and Post-Genocide Rwanda,*
https://doi.org/10.1007/978-3-030-74560-8_4

55

The concept of "marital happiness" indicates variables used in past research to measure satisfaction or happiness with various domains of the marriage (Dush et al., 2008). Marital happiness (Crohan & Veroff, 1989) as well as marital happiness and interaction (Johnson et al., 1986) have been conceptualized as among dimensions of marital quality. The quality of marriage has gained the attention of researchers (Bradbury et al., 2000; Nurhayati et al. 2019). Quality of marriage is defined in the literature as the level of excellence in marriage based on certain characteristics (Nurhayati et al., 2019). In addition to the need or theoretical progress in understanding the nature and determinants of marital satisfaction, Bradbury et al. (2000) call for research that links marital processes with socio-cultural contexts and for research that directly guides preventive, clinical, and policy-level interventions. Apart from marital happiness other dimensions of marital quality are marital conflict, marital commitment, social support, marital interaction, marital discord, forgiveness, and domestic violence (Stanley, 2007). It is suggested that the dimensions of marital quality vary widely, which can be distinguished into intrapersonal and interpersonal dimensions (Nurhayati et al., 2019).

Marital happiness is a judgment made by a spouse that indicates the sense of well being or satisfaction he or she experiences in the marital relationship (Fincham, 2009). Marital happiness is a critical element for the family life good functioning. Spouses who are satisfied in their marriage are also happy spouses (Fatima & Ajmal, 2012). People in happy marriages are able to think about their relationship differently from people in troubled marriages. Unhappily married people often hold their partner responsible for negative behaviors, but attribute positive behavior to other factors (Durtschi et al., 2011). Glenn and Weaver (1981) state that unmarried people are happier than people who are unhappily married and this is a good indicator of the importance of living happy marriage.

Satisfied spousal life is a happy marital life (Fatima & Ajmal, 2012). There is relationship between marital quality and health (Bookwala, 2005; Umberson et al., 2006). Marital quality affects the health impacts of marriage (Kiecolt-Glaser & Newton, 2001). Self-reported satisfaction with the relationship, low levels of hostile and negative behavior between spouses and positive attitudes toward one's spouse are characteristics of marital quality (Robles et al., 2014).

Marital happiness is an important indicator of marital quality (Dush et al., 2008). Marital happiness is a strong predictor of marital stability (White & Booth 1991). Marital quality is a determinant of psychological well-being (Davila et al., 1997; Dush et al., 2008; Frech & Williams, 2007; Kim & McKenry, 2002; Proulx et al., 2007). Coyne and Delongis (1986) suggest that an unhappy marriage is a significant source of stress. Low-quality marriages have significant negative effects on overall well-being (Hawkins & Booth, 2005; Whisman & Baucom, 2011). These authors (Hawkins & Booth, 2005; Whisman & Baucom, 2011) argue that staying unhappily married is more detrimental than divorcing, as people in low-quality marriages have lower levels of life satisfaction, self-esteem and overall health than individuals who remain unmarried.

Marital happiness as a dimension of marital quality is an essential element for successful family life and personal growth (Patel & Dhar, 2018). It indicates the sense of well-being or satisfaction experienced in the marital relationship (Patel & Dhar, 2018). A happy and prosperous married life is the ultimate goal for anyone who is either already married or is thinking about it (Murphy et al., 1997). The concept of marital quality can be different and can be developed in accordance to the local context (Nurhayati et al., 2019).

Determinants of Marital Happiness as a Dimension of Marital Quality in Ancient Rwandan Society

The outcomes presented in this chapter about the determinants of marital happiness as a dimension of marital quality in the pre-genocide Rwandan society are from the field data collected from Rwandan elders. These were distributed into a mixed group made up of 2 males and 3 females selected in the "guardian of memory" known as *Inteko Izirikana* (IN) located in Kigali city; a mixed group made up of 5 males and 2 females from Rwanda Elders Advisory Forum (RE) in

Kigali City; two homogeneous groups made of 7 Males and 11 Females respectively selected in the district of Nyanza (Ny) of the southern province of Rwanda; and two homogeneous groups made up of 8 Males and 7 Females respectively selected in the district of Karongi (Ka) of western province of Rwanda. The data were collected and analyzed using methodological approaches detailed in the chapter two titled "a qualitative research approaches to psychosocial well-being and mental health of individuals in marital and in family relationships in pre-post genocide Rwanda" of this book titled "psychosocial well-being and mental health of individuals in marital and in family relationships in pre-post genocide Rwanda".

In the pre-genocide Rwandan society, people would get married because of a number of reasons. These were the reasons of getting married (to have children, to increase the social support through the ties established between the two families, and to get and increase wealth); and the spousal marital life functioning (respect toward the in-law family members, communication and living peacefully, and mutual respect, love and balanced power relation coupled with a relations based on obeying each other).

Marital Happiness Was Linked to the Fulfillment of the Reasons of Getting Married in the Ancient Rwandan Society

As was mentioned by the participants in the present study, people in ancient Rwandan society would get married because they wanted to have children, to increase their social support through the ties established with the other family, to increase their own wealth, to have many cows and/or to have great harvest to put in the granaries as this could upgrade one's social class. So, whenever the spouses were in a situation where they felt that these reasons were fulfilled, they ought to happy in their marital life. The spousal happiness was linked to the fulfillment of the following reasons that prompt people to get married.

To Have Children

Happiness in the ancient Rwandan household was achieved when the couples were blessed with procreation. Children were seen as a blessing for a household. Having children was also seen as a way for the household to get more power and feel strengthened. Giving birth to children would not only bring happiness in the household, but it would as well confer value to the wife in the ancient Rwandan society. In the ancient Rwandan society, social life considered that giving birth was one of the ways to confer social consideration and value to the wife.

The blessed and happy household was one where there were children, and having children and raising them up was a source of pleasure in the household. (RE, Male). Giving birth conferred a social value to the wife. For a lady who, after marriage, had failed to give birth, one of her relatives could decide to give her one child so as to help her gain value in society. (IN, Female)

Human procreation is highly valued in African societies (Dhont et al., 2011). There was a profound conviction in African societies that children are a blessing for marriage and having children was a way of achieving a marriage objective (Chereji & King, 2015). Producing children during a marriage life was one of the common expectations and desire to achieve marital happiness. Having children was a source of happiness for the spouses in their marital life in the ancient Rwandan society. This is common in other African societies. Children secure conjugal ties, offer social security, confer social status, and satisfy emotional needs (Dyer, 2007). In a study conducted by VanLaningham et al. (2001), the respondents who had children were happier as compared to those who did not have any children, and the presence of children in the household was significantly related to marital happiness. Marriage and the presence of children in the household are determinants of marital happiness (Vanassche et al., 2013). The correlation between marital happiness and the presence of children in the household has been shown (Amato et al., 2007; Anderson et al., 1983; Vanassche et al., 2013).

To Increase Social Support Through the Ties Established Between the Two Families

Happiness in the ancient Rwandan households was brought by the fact that the two families unified through marriage were socially getting stronger thanks to these ties established between them. This was like having more social power rather than having one family not linked to others by the marriage. Making two different families of the couple closer to each other by marriage is one of the important aspects of the marriage (Fatima & Ajmal, 2012). Establishing ties between two families through the marriage of their two children was a way of socially strengthening each of those two families. This social support from the families to the new spouses was an important factor of happiness.

Marriage increases relationship and social support from the ties within the two families. Marriage itself is an important source of social support (Robles et al., 2014). The importance of marriage on health is that it creates social ties between two families and improves the social relationships and this benefits their health and well-being. It is suggested that social ties provide people with a sense of identity, purpose, belonging and support (Thoits, 2011). Marital happiness has been found to correlate with the interdependence of familial and friendship networks (Coombs, 1991; Kearns & Leonard, 2004; Zimmermann & Easterlin, 2006).

A happy and prosperous married life is the ultimate goal for anyone who is either already married or is thinking about it (Murphy et al., 1997). Satisfaction level decides one's level of happiness and, therefore, satisfied married life is considered as a happy married life (Fatima & Ajmal, 2012). A study conducted by Patel and Dhar (2018) revealed that marital happiness was seven times higher among married people who had high social support compared with those who had low social support. From the current study, we can say that the social support to married spouses in the ancient Rwandan society was a source of happiness as well as of well-being to them. Spousal social support is a social mechanism that might be responsible for marital outcomes (Fincham, 2003). The social support is one of the strong predictors for marital happiness (Patel & Dhar, 2018). Social support has a positive and highly significant association with marital happiness. The spouses who had higher social support have reported higher happiness (Van Laningham et al., 2001). Social support is one of the significant factors in marital relationships (Richter et al., 2014). The fulfillment and positive development will be possible only when the relationship between a couple is coherent and satisfactory (Abdul Azeez, 2013).

To Obtain and/or Increase Wealth

The spouses would feel some happiness when both of them could fulfill their respective responsibilities and give their respective contribution so as to make the household's economy and growth get bigger.

> Happiness was experienced in the household when each spouse fulfilled their own responsibilities well toward the household's economic growth. (Ka, Male).

> Happiness was in the household when the spouses collaborated to have wealth. (RE, Male)

The married people had to work to have wealth and wealth growth. They worked to have many cows if they were breeders and larger pieces of land for later huge harvests to put in the granaries if their source of income consisted in digging. They would work to increase their wealth so that they could upgrade their social class. Marital happiness correlates with household income (Kearns & Leonard, 2004). Marital happiness has been found to correlate with the household income (Amato et al., 2007).

To Abide by Cultural Conditions for Good Marital Life Functioning

The marital life functioning had various aspects, dictated by the culture. These aspects were related to the respect toward the in-law family members, collaboration of both spouses in contributing to the wealth of the household, good communication between spouses, common marital life direction, the mutual respect coupled with obeying each other, love and balanced power relation among the spouses, and living the marital life peacefully but to mention a few.

To Show Respect Toward the in-Law Family Members

In the ancient Rwandan society, the spouses would experience happiness when they felt that there was a culture of reciprocal respect of the in-law family members such as the brothers-in-law in their household. Each spouse was to respect the family members of his/her partner.

> The happiness would come from the culture of respect of the in-law family members for each one. When the brothers-in-law came to the new home and when they were respected. (Ny, Male)

While the importance of good relations with the in-laws could vary from a culture to another (Fatima & Ajmal, 2012; Patel & Dhar, 2018), these good relations were important in the marital life in ancient Rwandan society. They contributed to the spousal happiness as this was expressed by the elders, Rwandan nationals who participated in the present study. Quality of spouses' relationships with their parents-in-law would predict spouses' marital success; conflicts in extended family relations will erode marital stability, satisfaction, and commitment over time (Bryant et al., 2001).

To Maintain Good Communication and Live Together Peacefully

Communication between the spouses was an important key for happiness of the household's members. Good interactions in sitting together and discussing, sharing the meals and drinking while conversing with each other was a source of happiness in the household.

The household members would get happy sitting and discussing while they were eating and ultimately they would feel at ease. They used to drink milk together, and then they could get pleased. (Ka, Male)

What used to bring happiness in households was the time when the spouses were sitting down and conversing together. (Ny, Male)

Something which could make a happy household was good communication between the spouses and absence of negative disputation in the household. (Ny, Female)

Communication was a way of enabling the couple to have common marital direction, make same judgment and get same understanding regarding the household issues. Consequently, the fact of seeing everything in the same way, i.e. having an agreement on the household matters could make each other to get pleased. (RE, Male)

Communication and peaceful marital life as well as absence of negative disputation in the household was a source of marital happiness between the spouses. There is a positive correlation between marital satisfaction and communication (Ibrahimi & Jhanbozorgi, 2008). Communication leading to common marital life direction among the spouses was a source of happiness. Spouses were happy in ancient homes when they could communicate and when they had common understanding about their common journey in their marriage. Happiness was in the household when the spouses had the same judgment and could see what was happening in their home the same way.

To Safeguard Mutual Respect, Love, and Balanced Power Relations Coupled with Relations Based on Obeying Each Other

These behavioral values among the spouses were sources of happiness in the household in ancient Rwandan society. The household members would respect each other and live a harmonious life in their households and that life style was a source of happiness.

Being respected in the household and being proud of his wife or her husband helped the household members to be happy and live thinking that their home was peaceful. The wife would respect and make her husband be respected as a man among men so that people could say: [that man is dignified!]. The husband also had to respect and dignify his wife. For a spouse, the power was an important thing that was based on for one to be happy. In fact, the spouses, i.e. husband and wife, had the same power with regard to their property. For example, the husband could not give a cow to someone as a gift without his wife's consent and the wife could not distribute something in absence of her husband's consent. They both used to reach consensus on anything. (RE, Male)

Marital life, mutual respect among spouses was the cornerstone of the household happiness in the ancient Rwandan society. Such achieved marital life functioning was a subject of happiness for the household members and that was praised by the surrounding social environment as well. The married people had same materialistic power and reciprocal and mutual respect in their home and that power was one of the factors to confer happiness to them. The household members were happy to live together, to obey and to love each other and that was a source of happiness for the spouses. The coherence and satisfactory relationship between spouses make the achievement of positive development possible (Lawrence et al., 2019). Sharing power over decisions in marriage improves both the marriage and the individual psychological well-being (Dush et al., 2008). Marital happiness has been found to correlate with the egalitarian attitudes (Amato et al., 2007).

Conclusion

This chapter reports on the conditions of healthy marriage and of marital happiness in the households of the ancient Rwandan society. The conditions of happiness in marital homes of pre-genocide Rwandan society were closely related to the achievement of the reasons that make people get married as well as to the good spousal marital life functioning. For the marriage to bring happiness, there were some reasons and requirements to be met. These included having children, getting an increased social support through the ties established with the other family, experiencing an increase of own wealth. The conditions of happiness related to the spousal marital life functioning including respect toward the in-law family members, collaboration of both spouses in contributing to the increase of wealth of the household, good communication between spouses, common marital life direction, mutual respect coupled with obeying each other, love and balanced power relation among the spouses, and ultimately the living of marital life in a peaceful manner. The perceptions of the Rwandan Elders participants about the characteristics of marital life in traditional Rwandan society were not divergent based on any criteria such as gender or geographical location of the participants.

The findings presented in this chapter will be of interest for the following people but not limited to the policy makers and to the various practitioners in the field of mental health and psychosocial support. Even if data from focus group discussions may not be generalized, the cultural context of the current findings allow for an extendable insight from how marital life in the ancient Rwandan society went on and some experiences can be taken from there, built on and be adapted in home grown solution for a healthier marital life in today's Rwandan society. This means that today's marital life can improve, if policies makers and practitioners set innovative marriage mentor programs, marriage and family therapy structures, and continue preventive efforts toward marital satisfaction, happiness and family well-being for Rwandan community members.

Acknowledgements This research was conducted through the financial support of the University of Rwanda-Sweden Program.

Declaration of Interest Statement
There is no conflict of interest.

References

Abdul Azeez, E. P. (2013). Employed women and marital satisfaction: A study among female nurses. *International Journal of Management and Social Sciences Research, 2*(11), 17–26.

Amato, P. R., Booth, A., Johnson, D. R., & Rogers, S. J. (2007). *Alone together: How marriage in America is changing*. Harvard University Press.

Anderson, S. A., Russell, C. S., & Schumm, W. R. (1983). Perceived marital quality and family life-cycle categories: A further analysis. *Journal of Marriage and Family, 45*(1), 127–139. https://doi.org/10.2307/351301.

Argyle, M. (1999). Causes and correlates of happiness. In D. Kahneman, E. Diener, & N. Schwarz (eds.), *Well-being: The Foundations of Hedonic Psychology* (pp. 353–373). Russell Sage Foundation.

Bookwala, J. (2005). The role of marital quality in physical health during the mature years. *Journal of Aging and Health, 17*(1), 85–104. https://doi.org/10.1177/0898264304272794.

Bradbury, T. N., Fincham, F. D., & Beach, S. R. (2000). Research on the nature and determinants of marital satisfaction: A decade in review. *Journal of Marriage and Family, 62*(4), 964–980. https://doi.org/10.1111/j.1741-3737.2000.00964.x.

Bryant, C. M., Conger, R. D., & Meehan, J. M. (2001). The influence of in-laws on change in marital success. *Journal of Marriage and Family, 63*(3), 614–626. https://doi.org/10.1111/j.1741-3737.2001.00614.x.

Chereji, C.-R., & King, C. W. (2015). Aspects of traditional conflict management practices among the Ogoni of Nigeria. *Conflict Studies Quarterly, 10*, 56–68.

Coombs, R. H. (1991). Marital status and personal well-being: A literature review. *Family Relations: an Interdisciplinary Journal of Applied Family Studies, 40*(1), 97–102. https://doi.org/10.2307/585665.

Coyne, J. C., & DeLongis, A. (1986). Going beyond social support: The role of social relationships in adaptation. *Journal of Consulting and Clinical Psychology, 54*(4), 454–460. https://doi.org/10.1037/0022-006X.54.4.454.

Crohan, S. E., & Veroff, J. (1989). Dimensions of marital well-being among White and Black newlyweds. *Journal of Marriage and the Family, 51*(2), 373–383. https://doi.org/10.2307/352500.

Davila, J., Bradbury, T. N., Cohan, C. L., & Tochluk, S. (1997). Marital functioning and depressive symptoms: Evidence for a stress generation model.

Journal of Personality and Social Psychology, 73(4), 849–861. https://doi.org/ 10.1037/0022-3514.73.4.84.

Dhont, N., van de Wijgert, J., Coene, G., Gasarabwe, A., & Temmerman, M. (2011). "Mama and papa nothing": Living with infertility among an urban population in Kigali, Rwanda. *Human Reproduction, 26*(3), 623–629. https://doi.org/10.1093/humrep/deq373.

Dush, C. M. K., Taylor, M. G., & Kroeger, R. A. (2008). Marital Happiness And Psychological Well-Being Across The Life Course. *Family Relations, 57*(2), 211–226. https://doi.org/10.1111/j.1741-3729.2008.00495.x.

Durtschi, J. A., Fincham, F. D., Cui, M., Lorenz, F. O., & Conger, R. D. (2011). Dyadic processes in early marriage: Attributions, behavior, and marital quality. *Family Relations, 60*(4), 421–434. https://doi.org/10.1111/ j.1741-3729.2011.00655.x.

Dyer, S. J. (2007). The value of children in African countries: Insights from studies on infertility. *Journal of Psychosomatic Obstetrics & Gynecology, 28*(2), 69–77. https://doi.org/10.1080/01674820701409959.

Fatima, M., & Ajmal, M. A. (2012). Happy marriage: A qualitative study. *Pakistan Journal of Social and Clinical Psychology, 10*(1), 37–42.

Fincham, F. D. (2003). Marital conflict: Correlates, structure and context. *Current Directions in Psychological Science, 12*(23), 23–27. https://doi.org/ 10.1111/1467-8721.01215.

Fincham, F. D. (2009). *Marital happiness: The encyclopedia of positive psychology.* Blackwell.

Frech, A., & Williams, K. (2007). Depression and the psychological benefits of entering marriage. *Journal of Health and Social Behavior, 48*(2), 149–163. https://doi.org/10.1177/002214650704800204.

Glenn, N. D., & Weaver, C. N. (1981). The contribution of marital happiness to global happiness. *Journal of Marriage and Family., 43*(1), 161–168. https://doi.org/10.2307/351426.

Hawkins, D. N., & Booth, A. (2005). Unhappily Ever after: Effects of Long-Term, Low-Quality Marriages on Well-Being. *Social Forces, 84*(1), 451–471. https://doi.org/10.1353/sof.2005.0103.

Ibrahimi, A., & Jhanbozorgi, M. (2008). Relationship between communication skills and marital satisfaction. *Psychology and Religion, 1*(2), 147–164.

Johnson, D. R., White, L. K., Edwards, J. N., & Booth, A. (1986). Dimensions of marital quality: Toward methodological and conceptual refinement. *Journal of Family Issues, 7*(1), 31–49. https://doi.org/10.1177/019251386 007001003.

Kearns, J. N., & Leonard, K. E. (2004). Social networks, structural interdependence, and marital quality over the transition to marriage: a prospective analysis. *Journal of Family Psychology, 18*(2), 383–395. https://doi.org/10. 1037/0893-3200.18.2.383.

Kiecolt-Glaser, J. K., & Newton, T. L. (2001). Marriage and health: His and hers. *Psychological Bulletin, 127*(4), 472–503. https://doi.org/10.1037/ 0033-2909.127.4.472.

Kim, H. K., & McKenry, P. C. (2002). The relationship between marriage and psychological well-being: A longitudinal analysis. *Journal of Family Issues, 23*(8), 885–911. https://doi.org/10.1177/019251302237296.

Kushlev, K., Heintzelman, S. J., Lutes, L. D., Wirtz, D., Kanippayoor, J. M., Leitner, D., & Diener, E. (2020). Does happiness improve health? Evidence from a randomized controlled trial. *Psychological Science,* 1–15. https://doi. org/10.1177/0956797620919673.

Lavazza, A. (2016). Happiness, psychology, and degrees of realism. *Frontiers in Psychology, 7,* 1148. https://doi.org/10.3389/fpsyg.2016.01148.

Lawrence, E. M., Rogers, R. G., Zajacova, A., & Wadsworth, T. (2019). Marital happiness, marital status, health, and longevity. *Journal of Happiness Studies, 20*(5), 1539–1561. https://doi.org/10.1007/s10902-018-0009-9.

Murphy, M., Glaser, K., & Grundy, E. (1997). Marital status and long-term illness in Great Britain. *Journal of Marriage and the Family, 59*(1), 156–164. https://doi.org/10.2307/353669.

Nurhayati, S. R., Faturochman, F., & Helmi, A. K. (2019). Marital quality: A conceptual review. *Buletin Psikologi, 27*(2), 109–124. https://doi.org/10. 22146/buletinpsikologi.37691.

Patel, K. K., & Dhar, M. (2018). Marital happiness among newly married individuals in a rural district in India. *Social Science Spectrum, 4*(2), 76–85.

Proulx, C. M., Helms, H. M., & Buehler, C. (2007). Marital quality and personal well-being: A meta-analysis. *Journal of Marriage and Family, 69,* 576–593. https://doi.org/10.1111/j.1741-3737.2007.00393.x.

Richter, J., Rostami, A., & Ghazinour, M. (2014). Marital satisfaction, coping, and social support in female medical staff members in Tehran University Hospitals. *Interpersona: An International Journal on Personal Relationships, 8*(1), 115–127. https://doi.org/10.5964/ijpr.v8i1.139.

Robles, T. F., Slatcher, R. B., Trombello, J. M., & McGinn, M. M. (2014). Marital quality and health: A meta-analytic review. *Psychological Bulletin, 140*(1), 140–87. https://doi.org/10.1037/a0031859. PMC 3872512. PMID 23527470.

Spanier, G. B., & Lewis, R. A. (1980). Marital quality: A review of the seventies. *Journal of Marriage and Family, 4*(42), 825–839. https://www.jstor.org/stable/351827.

Stanley, S. M. (2007). Assessing couple and marital relationships: Beyond form and toward a deeper knowledge of function. In L. M. Casper, & S. L. Hoffereth (eds.), *Handbook of measurement issues in family research* (pp. 85–100). Lawrence Erlbaum & Associates.

Thoits, P. A. (2011). Mechanisms linking social ties and support to physical and mental health. *Journal of Health and Social Behavior, 52*(2), 145–161. https://doi.org/10.1177/0022146510395592.

Umberson, D., Williams, K., Powers, D. A., Liu, H., & Needham, B. (2006). You make me sick: Marital quality and health over the life course. *Journal of Health and Social Behavior, 47*, 1–16. https://doi.org/10.1177/002214650 604700101.

Vanassche, S., Swicegood, G., & Matthijs, K. (2013). Marriage and children as a key to happiness? Cross-national differences in the effects of marital status and children on well-being. *Journal of Happiness Studies, 14*, 501–524. https://doi.org/10.1007/s10902-012-9340-8.

VanLaningham, J., Johnson, D. R., & Amato, P. (2001). Marital happiness, marital duration, and the U-shaped curve: Evidence from a five-wave panel study. *Social Forces, 79*(4), 1313–1341. https://doi.org/10.1353/sof.2001. 0055.

Whisman, M. A., & Baucom, D. H. (2011). Intimate relationships and psychopathology. *Clinical Child and Family Psychology Review, 15*(1), 4–13. https://doi.org/10.1007/s10567-011-0107-2.

White, L. K., & Booth, A. (1991). Divorce over the life course: The role of marital happiness. *Journal of Family Issues, 12*, 5–21. https://doi.org/10. 1177/019251391012001002.

Zimmermann, A., & Easterlin, R. A. (2006). Happily ever after? Cohabitation, marriage, divorce and happiness in Germany. *Population and Development Review, 32*, 511–528. https://doi.org/10.1111/j.1728-4457.2006.00135.x.

5

Socio-Cultural Causes of Marriage Destruction in Ancient Rwandan Society

Immaculée Mukashema, Joseph Gumira Hahirwa, Alexandre Hakizamungu, and Lambert Havugintwari

Introduction

Conflict is a natural and inherent phenomena in marital relations, as a result of different interests, opinions, and perspectives between couple members (Delatorre & Wagner, 2018). Marital conflict was conceptualized as an overt opposition between spouses, which generates disagreements and relationship difficulties (Fincham, 2009).

Marital conflict may be constructive or destructive (Goeke-Morey et al., 2003; McCoy et al., 2009). Marital conflict is said to be constructive when spouses deal with conflict in positive ways by displaying behaviors, such as verbal and physical affection, problem solving and support (McCoy et al., 2009; Goeke-Morey et al., 2003). Marital conflict is described as destructive when it is hostile, angry, and contains conflict tactics such as physical aggression, verbal aggression, threat, and personal

I. Mukashema (✉) · J. Gumira Hahirwa · A. Hakizamungu · L. Havugintwari
College of Arts and Social Sciences, University of Rwanda, Butare, Rwanda

© The Author(s), under exclusive license to Springer Nature Switzerland AG 2021
I. Mukashema (ed.), *Psychosocial Well-Being and Mental Health of Individuals in Marital and in Family Relationships in Pre- and Post-Genocide Rwanda*,
https://doi.org/10.1007/978-3-030-74560-8_5

insult (McCoy et al., 2009; Goeke-Morey et al., 2003). There is a link between marital problems and mental illness (Fincham, 2003; Kiecolt-Glaser & Newton, 2001; Robles et al., 2014; Whisman & Baucom, 2011)

The problem of destructive marital conflict has not yet been sufficiently explored in Rwanda (Mukashema & Sapsford, 2013). The small number of publications available cover a period referred to as the post-genocide period in Rwanda. It is noted that the genocide of 1994 perpetrated against the Tutsis is a reference time separating the pre- and post-periods in relation to that genocide. As a matter of fact, the genocide had several consequences, including psychosocial ones. In this perspective, marital conflict in Rwanda can be seen as a legacy of that genocide (Sarabwe et al., 2018). Other mentioned causes of the alarming destructive marital conflict in Rwanda today include misinterpretation of gender-related laws by spouses (Ndushabandi et al., 2016) as well as a misunderstanding of gender roles and human rights (Mukashema & Sapsford, 2013).

The contribution of this chapter is that it describes the elders' views on socio-cultural causes of marriage destruction in the traditional Rwandan society. The chapter is an attempt toward devising a possible solution to the alarming state of marital and family life today through a Rwandan cultural lens.

Socio-Cultural Causes of Marriage Destruction in the Ancient Rwandan Society

The outcomes presented in this chapter about the characteristics of marital and family life in customary Rwanda are from the field data collected from Rwandan elders. These participants were distributed in a mixed group made up of two males and three females selected from the "Guardian of memory" known as *Inteko Izirikana* (IN) located in Kigali city; a mixed group made up of five males and two females from the Rwanda Elders Advisory Forum (RE) in Kigali City; two homogeneous groups made up of seven males and eleven females respectively, selected from the district of Nyanza (Ny) of the southern province of Rwanda;

and two homogeneous groups made up of eight males and seven females respectively, selected from the district of Karongi (Ka) of the western province of Rwanda.

The data were collected and analyzed using methodological approaches detailed in Chapter 2 of this book.

The findings reveal that there was destructive marital conflict in pre-genocide Rwandan society. The causes of marriage destruction in ancient Rwandan society as voiced by the research participants included: hidden disease and malformation, adultery, marital sexual relation dissatisfaction, uncleanliness and lack of hygiene on the side of the wife, drunkenness, disrespect, stealing, and infertility.

Existence or Non-existence of Destructive Marital Conflict in Pre-genocide Rwandan Society

Destructive marital conflict is the key focus of this research. With reference to the general tendency in the views of Rwandan elders who participated in the study, destructive marital conflict existed in pre-genocide Rwandan society.

> Marital conflict existed and there is no doubt about this. If a woman could leave her husband and flee the marital home, this is a strong evidence that conflicts between her and her husband existed. Psychological and even physical violence existed too. Spouses could repeatedly exchange negative words, a situation of discussions which was not aimed at solutions to problems but rather a mere dispute which could lead to the spouses fighting among themselves. (RE, male)

> I confirm marital conflict existed and that its causes were numerous. For example, marital conflict could result from behavior like exaggerated drunkenness. However, let's remember that the families had a way of preparing the future spouses to show good behaviors and patience with each other. In some instances, a woman could be beaten by her husband to mean that domestic violence and marital conflict existed. (RE, female)

Destructive marital conflict existed in ancient Rwandan society but that was not so frequent. The participants in the study made it clear that there could be some marital conflict cases among the ancient Rwandan spouses, but added that conflict was not really frequent. Destructive marital conflict could occur in ancient Rwandan society, but it was not frequent. (RE, female)

There could be destructive marital conflict cases in the ancient Rwandan society, but they were not frequent. They were not so many cases of conflict which could be noticed. I can say that you could hardly see very few spouses in marital quarrel in ancient Rwanda. (Ny, female)

Conflict was not inexistent among rational Rwanda spouses, but it would not often spread to the public to be known to all. (Ny, male)

Marital conflicts existed but there were mechanisms to prevent and resolve them in order to sustain marital homes. In short, marital conflict existed. (RE, female)

The difference between Rwandan ancient marital homes and those of today is that in ancient Rwandan society, there were cultural safeguards which would push the spouses to get rid of situations of shame such as marital conflict. Marital secrecy was primarily a value that was preserved and this would make the spouses handle the disputes internally. Each spouse would try their best to avoid disappointment to their extended families of origin. Today, however, there is no place for the family, the spouses are individualistic. (IN, male)

The spouses in ancient Rwandan society would discuss and agree on everything to do in the marital home. I, myself, can confirm that from time to time, there was some little conflict between my own parents but we could not get to know anything about this as children. We cannot say that there was no conflict between the parents, but the parents could not argue in the eyes of their children. (IN, female)

In ancient Rwandan society, there were cultural ways of preventing destructive marital conflict in new households. The prevention of destructive marital conflict in new households would mainly and primarily run through the family upbringing of the children and youth. Firstly, the children were to observe the parental life process, and secondly they would abide by the verbal pieces of advice given to them especially just before the time of their own marriage. In ancient Rwandan society, the parental marital daily lifestyle was playing an important role in preventing destructive marital conflict for the future spouses. It was a kind of training based on a family life approach aiming at the preparation of young people to their marriage in future and to their subsequent marital life. (IN, female)

The young people would observe their parents living carefully and peacefully in their own marital life. This could serve as a lesson and help them such that they would also avoid destructive marital conflict when they get married. (RE, Male)

The destructive marital conflict prevention was also done through verbal pieces of advice which specifically were given to the young people about to get married. They would be guided on the action to be taken in case of conflict in their new household. In their respective family of origin, the bride and the groom, through observation, would learn and get prepared for their marriage. They would be told that if a controversy rises in their life once married, they ought not to fight each other. They would rather have to approach the parents and tell them what was going wrong. The parents would then help them manage the controversial situations. (Ny, female)

Causes of Marriage Destruction in the Ancient Rwandan Society

In the ancient Rwandan society, the factors of marriage destruction included diseases, disabilities, and misbehaviors. As a result of one or combination of these, there could be separation of the spouses, thus marriage destruction. The participants in this research stressed a number of misbehaviors on the side of the spouses that were taken as a very serious and particular offence, especially when they were exhibited by women. They also highlighted some other causes that could lead to marital conflict that include the following.

Hidden Disease and Physical Malformation

In the ancient Rwandan society, it was a taboo for the prospective spouses to have sex before marriage. They would meet for the first time on the very day of their marriage. Because of this practice in the marriage process, it was possible for a spouse to discover a given abnormality in his/her partner. That abnormality could be a physical abnormality or a hidden disease. Depending on the type of abnormality, it was possible that the marriage could end there. If abnormality was noticed on the side of the wife, she was sent back to her family of origin (*gusenda*). If, however it was noticed in the husband, he was left by his wife. The ancient Rwandan society was of the view that there was nothing wrong in doing so in such a situation.

> As the spouses could not know each other before their marriage, it was possible that either of them might discover an abnormality in the other and that abnormality could make the marriage end immediately. The wife was sent back to her family of origin (*gusenda*), the husband was left by his wife because the society was viewing this as a right thing to do in case of abnormality or disease. A visible physical malformation or a hidden disease like tuberculosis would also be a cause of divorce. There was nothing wrong for a spouse to leave his/her partner in such a situation. (RE, male)

> If a woman got married to a man and she found that the husband had a sickness like stinking (*isundwe*), then it was her right to leave that gentleman for good. (IN, male)

Adultery

If one of the spouses was ever engaged in some cheating, this could end in marriage break-up. Cases of adultery which had come to be known by the public could lead to the complete destruction of the marriage. Adultery, especially when committed by the wife, was particularly taken as an unforgivable sin.

If the husband was caught committing adultery for nearly two times, and when his wife had come to know it, this would eventually end up into marriage ruin. It was particularly a big shame for a wife who committed adultery though. When it was known that a wife had committed adultery, that behavior would make the husband kick his wife away to her family of origin or he would immediately leave her alone. The wife's adultery in the knowledge of the husband was such an unforgivable sin that it would cause a serious quarrel with him. (RE, male)

When a wife tended visibly to be attracted by other men, this tendency could also lead to the ruin of her marriage. (Ny, female)

Marital Sexual Relations Dissatisfaction

Sexual relations dissatisfaction could lead to marital disputes, which in turn could result in destructive marital conflict.

Sexual relations dissatisfaction could lead to marital disputes. When one of the spouses was not satisfied and felt displeased toward his/her partner, one of them, especially the dissatisfied one, could engage in some cheating and this could end in marriage break-up. (Ny, male)

A woman could be sent home by her husband on the ground of sexual dissatisfaction for the latter (RE, female)

Uncleanliness and Lack of Hygiene on the Side of the Wife

In the ancient Rwandan societies' gender roles, the wife was specifically in charge of the hygiene of the household, and for the hygiene of the members of her household, among other responsibilities.

When the wife was dirty and was failing to fulfill her responsibilities regarding assurance of proper hygiene in the household, this was a cause of marriage destruction. A wife with dirtiness was a case of humiliation for the family; this was an unbearable misbehavior. Dirtiness, i.e., lack of hygiene, was one of the causes of quarrel between spouses. (IN, male)

Drunkenness

Drunkenness on the side of the wife was not socially tolerated. It would cause quarrels between her and her husband unless the husband was too soft.

> Drunkenness was a misbehavior that could cause quarrels among spouses. When the wife was a drunkard, this was particularly serious and it was socially intolerable. There were bad behaviors which men could show and yet that the society could tolerate but it was so unlikely when it came to their wives. (IN, male)

Disrespect

The wife had to be careful about her behavior and ought to show a behavior of respect toward her husband.

> Whenever a husband had tried to make a call to his wife and yet the latter had neglected or refused to serve him as he had asked, that could lead to her expulsion from the family. Such behavior was more seriously castigated when efforts had been made for some time to correct her, but in vain. In this case, the husband would have a right to remarry with hope that the new wife could behave and show more respect to him than the first one. (Ny, female)

> When a husband had made allegations that his wife was showing disrespect toward him, this could have a lot of meaning in ancient Rwandan culture. For example, that would mean that when he returned home drunk, his wife maybe did not receive him with respect. It could mean also that things had not happen so properly in bed for him to obtain satisfaction. (RE, female)

Stealing

The act of stealing carried out by one of the spouses could be a possible reason to raise up conflict and lead to marriage destruction, and this misbehavior was mainly shown by men.

> When the husband was stealing the household property; i.e., if farm harvests were being dilapidated and/or taken away by the husband without any reason, and when this was noticed by the wife, this could lead to marriage break-up. (Ny, male)

Infertility

Failure to give birth in the household was attributed to the wife, and that was taken as an abnormality in the ancient Rwandan culture. As a result of this, the wife could be sent back to her family of origin.

> Among the abnormalities in ancient Rwandan society, there was infertility that would often be attributed to the woman who had failed to give birth. In such a situation, her husband could kick her out of the house and send her back to her family of origin. (RE, male)

> The woman could be sent home by her husband on the ground of infertility [here this does not say that there was evidence that it was the woman who was sterile]. (RE, female)

Discussion

This section discusses the findings regarding the views of the elders about the existence of destructive marital conflict and the causes of marriage destruction in the ancient Rwandan society. The findings show that even for the rare cases of destructive marital conflict which existed, the marital life shaping in ancient Rwandan society was such that there were mechanisms to deal with the spousal disputes within the families so as to avoid divorce. Divorce was socially allowed only for specific cases.

Existence or Non-existence of Destructive Marital Conflict in Ancient Rwandan Society

The existence of cases of destructive marital conflict was a reality in ancient Rwandan society, according to the participants in the current research. The findings illustrate that marital conflict is obviously a phenomenon that cannot totally be prevented by spouses. Marital conflict is linked to marital relations (Delatorre & Wagner, 2018; Fincham & Beach, 1999). Spouses in ancient Rwandan society did not make an exception to this, but cases of destructive marital conflict are said to have been not frequent. The concept of "non-frequency" with regard to marital conflict in ancient Rwandan society can actually be nuanced. This can be interpreted and/or explained in two ways.

On the one hand, one may assume that conflict existed and was probably frequent, but that it was not reported, or not easily discovered to become publicly known. Cultural values in ancient Rwanda were shaped in such a way that neither of the spouses would make their marital conflict publicaly known, i.e., revealed to the world outside their household and/or outside their two families of origin. This was learned naturally and by emulation from one generation to another, i.e., from parents to children, and the practice of keeping family business private was seriously stressed on prior to marriage.

On the other hand, the frequency of destructive marital conflict was really low because of permanent ties between new spouses and their families of origin. These two families of the spouses' origin had important roles to play in supporting the new spouses' good marital relations (Chereji & King, 2015). Participation and involvement of the spouses' families of origin, if not a constant presence, in the whole marriage process and during the marital life of the children, would somewhat constitute a cultural and psychosocial pressure to the new households. As a result of such pressure, the two spouses had to strive to prevent destructive marital conflict. This was triggered by the fact that marriage was seen as a union of the two in-law families beyond the fact of being a union between the two new spouses (Arugu, 2014). Thus, any misunderstanding between the spouses, which eventually could lead to the breach of such a union, would be a shame for their families (Chereji & King,

2015). Each of the spouses would do anything to prevent conflict for fear of creating public shame, not only on themselves, but also on the families they had been brought up in.

Causes of Marriage Destruction in the Ancient Rwandan Society

The Rwandans participating in this study did not mention marital conflict as a potential cause of marriage destruction as such in the ancient Rwandan society. Instead, they listed a number of factors which could lead to marital dissolution, i.e., marriage destruction, in ancient Rwanda. These factors of marriage destruction included hidden diseases, disabilities, and misbehaviors. The participants stressed misbehavior in spouses as very serious and particular offences, especially when they were exhibited by women.

Prior to marriage in some African traditional societies, investigation was conducted in order to find whether there existed various chronic diseases, especially the contagious ones, and to inquire about the behaviors in the family intended to become the family-in-law (Chereji & King, 2015). The investigation was necessary in order to protect and maintain the marriage and the moral status of the families as the family unit was the guarantor of security (Huyse & Salter, 2008). Sometimes, it was not easy to get to know about a disease in a spouse if this was not revealed, and the partner would later on be allowed to divorce if ever this was discovered.

When talking about spousal misbehaviors, the Rwandan elders participating in this study showed that some behaviors were specific to either sex. Bad behaviors like adultery were common to both wives and husbands. Some others like dirtiness and disrespect were considered bad behaviors exclusively in women; while stealing and the like could be particularly seen in men. Cases of adultery that had already come to be known by the public in the ancient Rwandan society could put an end to the marriage. When adultery was particularly committed by the wife, this was taken as an unforgivable sin. There was a mere exaggeration of women's adultery over men's, since adultery was a somewhat commonly tolerated practice. Research has shown that the culture could not tolerate the fact that someone's wife had committed adultery, and yet she still had further conjugal relations (Mathebula, 2017).

In a study conducted by Dhont et al. (2011), sexual relations dissatisfaction was more frequently reported by infertile than fertile couples. The psychosocial consequences suffered by infertile couples in Rwanda are severe and similar to those reported in other resource-poor countries (Dhont et al., 2011). When the wife was dirty or had failed to care for hygiene in the household, this was a cause of sending her back to her family of origin. Drunkenness displayed by a woman would cause quarrels between her and with her husband except when the latter was too soft. Also, researchers suggest that an African man is likely to divorce his wife when he feels that she disrespects him (Preller, 2014; Scarpitti & Anderson, 2011).

Infertility was a cause of marriage break-up in ancient Rwandan society. The absence of fertility was attributed to the wife. In African societies in general, there was a profound conviction that children are a blessing, and so failure to produce children was considered a misfortune. There is a belief that a marriage without children has not yet achieved its objectives (Chereji & King, 2015). A marriage that is not blessed with children has not achieved its aim (Arugu, 2014). Infertile women were more likely to encounter domestic violence (Rahebi et al., 2019). Traditionally, the state of childlessness in marriage within some African societies was a factor that could influence and lead to automatic divorce (Chereji & King, 2015). A childless marriage could be a cause of divorce in the ancient Rwandan society as well.

Conclusion

This research verified the existence of destructive marital life and described the causes of marriage destruction in ancient Rwandan society. Marital conflict existed in ancient Rwandan society but cases were not frequent or alarming. This can have a double explanation. First, there were cultural values that would stop the spouses from making marital conflicts publicly known. Second, marital conflict in new homes within ancient Rwandan society was prevented through an upbringing from a young age that would lead to some emulation of the parents. New spouses would behave in the ways they had observed throughout the marital life course of their parents, and would go by the advice given to them by their elders, prior to their marriage.

Even if divorce was not seen as an option to solve marital problems in the ancient Rwandan society, there were culturally accepted cases where the spouses were allowed to divorce. These included: cases of adultery, discovering of a hidden disease or/and malformation in one of the spouses, marital sexual relations dissatisfaction, dirtiness and lack of hygiene on the side of the wife, drunkenness, disrespect, stealing, and infertility. Among the causes of marriage destruction in ancient Rwandan society, some seem to have been specific to either sex. Bad behaviors like adultery were common to both wives and husbands. Some others like dirtiness and disrespect were specifically considered for women, while stealing and the like could be particularly seen in men. Coping strategies in traditional Rwandan society should be explored, and the applicability of cultural values in preventing destructive marital conflict that has become frequent in today's new homes, is today essential.

Implications

The current research used focus group discussions, and thus the findings may not be generalized. However, they give insight on what marital life in the ancient Rwandan society was like, and some experiences can be taken from there, built on, and adapted to home-grown solutions for a better and healthier marital life in today's Rwandan society. The findings will be of particular interest for the following groups of people: participants in the current study, young people about to get married, policymakers, religious authorities, and married people.

Limitations

This chapter discussed the perceptions of participants on destructive marital conflict in ancient Rwandan society, and its goal has been achieved. However, applying it to the broader population would need further researches. The next researches could aim to systematically compare ancient and modern marital life in Rwandan society with a larger sample, and to explore the applicability of cultural values in preventing destructive marital conflict in today's new families.

Acknowledgements This research was conducted through the financial support of the University of Rwanda-Sweden Program.

Declaration of Interest Statement
There is no conflict of interest.

References

Arugu, L. O. (2014). Social indicators and effects of marriage divorce in African societies. *The Business & Management Review, 4*(4), 374–383.

Chereji, C.-R., & King, C. W. (2015). Aspects of traditional conflict management practices among the Ogoni of Nigeria. *Conflict Studies Quarterly, 10,* 56–68.

Delatorre, M. Z., & Wagner, A. (2018). Marital conflict management of married men and women. *Psico-USF, 23* (2). https://doi.org/10.1590/1413-82712018230204.

Dhont, N., van de Wijgert, J., Coene, G., Gasarabwe, A., & Temmerman, M. (2011). Mama and papa nothing: Living with infertility among an urban population in Kigali. *Rwanda. Human Reproduction, 26* (3), 623–629. https://doi.org/10.1093/humrep/deq373.

Fincham, F. D. (2003). Marital conflict: Correlates, structure and context. *Current Directions in Psychological Science, 12*(23), 23–27. https://doi.org/10.1111/1467-8721.01215.

Fincham, F. D. (2009). *Marital conflict: Encyclopedia of human relationships* (Vol. 1, pp. 298–303). Sage.

Fincham, F. D., & Beach, S. R. (1999). Marital conflict: Implications for working with couples. *Annual Review of Psychology, 50,* 47–77. https://doi.org/10.1146/annurev.psych.50.1.47.

Goeke-Morey, M. C., Cummings, E. M., Harold, G. T., & Shelton, K. H. (2003). Categories and continua of destructive and constructive marital conflict tactics from the perspective of U.S. and Welsh children. *Journal of Family Psychology, 17*(3),327–338. https://doi.org/10.1037/0893-3200.17.3.327.

Huyse, L., & Salter, M. (2008). *Traditional justice and reconciliation after violent conflict: Learning from African experiences.* International Institute for Democracy and Electoral Assistance (IDEA), Stockholm. https://www.idea.int/sites/default/files/publications/traditional-justice-and-reconciliation-after-violent-conflict-learning-from-african-experiences_0.pdf.

Kiecolt-Glaser, J. K., & Newton, T. L. (2001). Marriage and health: His and hers. *Psychological Bulletin, 127*(4), 472–503. https://doi.org/10.1037/0033-2909.127.4.472.

Mathebula, T. S. (2017). *Socio-behavioural and structural core drivers of new HIV infections in the Department of Agriculture, Mopani District of the Limpopo Province.* University of Limpopo. http://ulspace.ul.ac.za/bitstream/handle/10386/2058/mathebula_ts_2018.pdf?sequence=1&isAllowed=y.

McCoy, K., Cummings, E. M., & Davies, P. T. (2009). Constructive and destructive marital conflict, emotional security and children's prosocial behavior. *Journal of Child Psychology and Psychiatry, 50*(3), 270–279. https://doi.org/10.1111/j.1469-7610.2008.01945.x.

Mukashema, I., & Sapsford, R. (2013). Marital conflicts in Rwanda: Points of view of Rwandan psycho-socio-medical professionals. *Procedia-Social and Behavioral Sciences, 82*(2013), 149–168. https://doi.org/10.1016/j.sbspro.2013.06.239.

Ndushabandi, E. N., Kagaba, M., & Gasafari, W. (2016). *Intra-family conflicts in Rwanda: A constant challenge to sustainable peace in Rwanda.* http://www.irdp.rw/wp-content/uploads/2019/02/intrafamily-conflicts-last-version-2.pdf.

Preller, B. (2014). *Everyone's guide to divorce and separation.* Zebra Press.

Rahebi, S. M., Rahnavardi, M., Rezaie-Chamani, S., Nazari, M., & Sabetghadam, S. (2019). Relationship between domestic violence and infertility. *Eastern Mediterranean Health Journal, 25*(8), 537–542. https://doi.org/10.26719/emhj.19.001.

Robles, T. F., Slatcher, R. B., Trombello, J. M., & McGinn, M. M. (2014). Marital quality and health: A meta-analytic review. *Psychological Bulletin, 140*(1), 140–187. https://doi.org/10.1037/a0031859.

Sarabwe, E., Richters, A., & Vysma, M. (2018). Marital conflict in the aftermath of genocide in Rwanda: An explorative study within the context of community based sociotherapy. *Intervention, 16*(1), 14–21. https://doi.org/10.1097/WTF.0000000000000147.

Scarpitti, M., & Anderson, P. R. (2011). *Causes of divorce*. Allyn and Bacon.

Whisman, M. A., & Baucom, D. H. (2011). Intimate relationships and psychopathology. *Clinical Child and Family Psychology Review, 15*(1): 4–13. https://doi.org/10.1007/s10567-011-0107-2. PMID 22124792.

6

Protective Factors of Marriage Lastingness in Traditional Rwandan Society

Immaculée Mukashema, Joseph Gumira Hahirwa, Alexandre Hakizamungu, and Lambert Havugintwari

Introduction

Marriage is seen as a long-term commitment (Lauer & Lauer, 1986; Swensen & Trahaug, 1985). For happy couples, the most frequently named reasons given in a research for staying together, are the perceived nature of the relationship, the belief in marriage as a long-term commitment, and mutual devotion and special regard for each other among spouses (Lauer & Lauer, 1986). Explaining marriage lastingness in the psychodynamic perspective, Quinn (2019) argues that the final desirable feature of marriage is motivated by the infant's desire not to be abandoned, thus bringing in the spouses' best efforts, jointly and separately, to overcome marital incompatibility and bring about sufficient compatibility to make the marriage last. For unhappy marriages, the most frequently named reason for staying together was the belief that

I. Mukashema (✉) · J. Gumira Hahirwa · A. Hakizamungu ·
L. Havugintwari
College of Arts and Social Sciences, University of Rwanda, Butare, Rwanda

© The Author(s), under exclusive license to Springer Nature
Switzerland AG 2021
I. Mukashema (ed.), *Psychosocial Well-Being and Mental Health of Individuals in Marital and in Family Relationships in Pre- and Post-Genocide Rwanda*,
https://doi.org/10.1007/978-3-030-74560-8_6

marriage is a long-term commitment (Lauer & Lauer, 1986). Quinn (1996) states that lastingness is a property of a successful marriage. The author adds that all successful marriages are lasting ones, but that not all lasting marriages are successful. Quinn (1996) confirms that there exist "unhappy" lasting marriages.

This chapter explores the protective factors of marriage lastingness in ancient Rwanda. It comes from a broader research on the characteristics of marital and family life in customary Rwanda using Rwandan elders as participants. These participants in the research are as following: a mixed group made up of two males and three females selected in the "Guardian of memory" known as *Inteko Izirikana* (IN) located in Kigali city; a mixed group made up of five males and two females from Rwanda Elders Advisory Forum (RE) in Kigali City; two homogeneous groups made up of seven males and eleven females respectively, selected in the district of Nyanza (Ny) of the southern province of Rwanda; and two homogeneous groups made up of eight males and seven females respectively, selected in the district of Karongi (Ka) in the western province of Rwanda.

The data were collected and analyzed using methodological approaches detailed in Chapter 2 of this volume.

Marriage lastingness was possible mainly due to the psychosocial consideration of the families of origin in the new spouses' marital life, and to the roles that the spouses themselves had to play in safeguarding their marriage. The couples would make it possible through mutual respect between the spouses, and commitment of the spouses to marital life up to the "sacrifice" of living in conjugal trouble and stress in order to protect their marriage, and especially the well-being of the children. Patience and perseverance for marriage were key factors for a strong household.

The Psychosocial Consideration of the Families of Origin in the New Spouses' Marital Life

When two people got married in traditional Rwandan society, the marriage would serve some other purposes than just the interests of the spouses. The couple had the responsibility of being the bridge unifying their two families of origin. In other words, marriage was not an exclusive business of the spouses in traditional Rwanda. Marriage, instead, was for the interest of the two spouses' families of origin at large. The spouses were there to serve as ambassadors of their respective families of origin in the family of the in-laws.

> I would like to say that one of the married partners is not in marriage relationship for his or her own purpose; he/she is rather his/her family's ambassador in the in-law family. (REAF, female)

> Look at my age, but I am lucky to have my mother who is now 80–90 years old. I have asked her if everything was flawless in her matrimonial home. She told me no. She gave me an example of one of the times when her husband was tough on her and she told him she was going to go back to her parents. At this point, the husband made an effort to change for fear of being looked down upon by their two family members if ever his wife was to return to her parents. Spouses lived by pursuing the honor of their families, men sought the honor of their matrimonial homes, their wives. Wives could be patient even in conflict with her husband for the sake of protecting their children so that nothing bad would happen to them if she leaves them alone. (IN, female)

> When the two young people, a boy and a girl, were old enough to be married, their respective parents had the responsibilities of advising them on behaviors they would have to display in their marital life. These behaviors, among others, included good representation of their own family of origin in the family-in-law. The spouses had to be always careful and protect the ties established between their two families of origin. Each spouse was his/her family's ambassador for the in-law family. So, he/she had to do everything carefully so as not to be the reason of destroying anything about the two families' relationship. (REAF, female)

> The father and the mother used to tell the girl: "Listen, please, our beloved child; do not indecently represent us in that home you are going to make." The son was asked to take good care of his wife: "Take care of this woman, your wife; do not indecently represent us in that family [the bride's family of origin]." (REAF, male)

In traditional Rwanda, the new spouses had the psychosocial task of representing their family of origin in the family in-law very well. They had the psychosocial responsibility to unify their two families of origin and to protect the ties established between them. [...]

You had to unite your father-in-law and your born-home's family members. The new household intermediated both families. The spouses had to be the cornerstone support in the unity of both their families of origin. (REAF, male)

If you were a wife, you had to live so that both your family-in-law and your family of origin could live together in harmony; even when you were a husband, you had to unite your family-in-law and your born-home's family members. The new home intermediates for both families. (REAF, male)

Spouses had a psychosocial responsibility to prevent breakage of the family ties established between their two families of origin through their marriage. In a situation of marital problems, the spouses were required to find solutions without harming the relationship of their two families of origin. [...] the spouses had to be patient and had to have effective particular ways of solving problems without harming ties and relationship established between their families of origin. (REAF, female)

Each of the two spouses had the moral and psychosocial responsibility to avoid being the cause of the two families' separation or break-up of the ties and relationships established.

[...] For those who were married to each other, you had to not be the reason of the separation and the breaking of the ties and relationship established between their two families. They had to be careful about those two families, thinking: "What will my family of origin say...what will they comment on about it (my behavior)...As the married couple, there were some things you had to pay attention to in order not to make your family feel ashamed; you had to pay attention to your family of origin and your family-in-law's established ties. (REAF, male)

Marriage in traditional Rwanda was a matter of families' consensus (NISR, 2012). The marriage was considered a social obligation for each man and woman vis-à-vis their family in order to perpetuate the lineage (NISR, 2012). Before marriage, the two families had to play an important role in advising their young children about to get married on what their daily marriage life would be like. The purpose of the families' involvement was to help the young spouses to have a good marital life. Additionally, this involvement would make the new couple bear in mind the importance of keeping their two families of origin in good relations. This responsibility of being the "family's ambassador in the in-law family" would put the new spouses in a situation of living their marital life carefully. The new spouses had the psychosocial responsibility of protecting the established relationships and ties. Traditional marriages provided two primary advantages over any other relationships; and that was safety and stability (*The New Times*, 2007).

The Rwandan traditional spouses had the psychosocial responsibility of ensuring cohesion of their respective families of origin. Marriage in traditional Rwanda was a serious family matter. Marriage is not just a business of the couple concerned, it concerns all and is affected by all (Thompson, 2017). Marriage was an affiance, an agreement or contract between two families or groups of kin, because African societies see marriage not only as a relationship between two individual people but also as a structural link between groups (Thompson, 2017).

The Roles of Spouses Themselves in Safeguarding Their Marriage Lastingness

In traditional Rwandan society, spouses were characterized by mutual respect in their marital lives. Even in a situation of marital-life difficulties, the spouses could sacrifice themselves by continuing to live in that situation, and to be patient and tolerant to each other. This was the custom, and the ultimate goal behind this was the fear of making their children victims of marital break-up or social shame. In this sense, the presence of children in the household was a factor of lastingness. Bachand and Caron (2001) suggest that children play a key role in long-term marriages. The marriage could benefit from this commitment of protecting the children from suffering. Spouses who commit to marriage consider themselves to be a pair with a common future, and make further efforts to preserve their identity as a couple (Karimi et al., 2019). Commitment to marriage is an important factor for marriage lastingness. Commitment is conceptualized as the commitment to relationship, namely, the intent to persist in marriage (Le & Agnew, 2003; Tzitzika et al., 2020), and the wish to remain in the marriage even when confronted with difficulties (Schoebi et al., 2012). Spouses committed to marriage believe that they have to work out and solve their problems (Stanley et al., 2010).

Mutual Respect Between the Spouses

The spouses were characterized by mutual respect in their marital life. Consequently, their children would emulate and do the same later on once married.

> The spouses really respected each other: the husband respected the wife and the wife respected the husband. Therefore, they would seek for a affordable way of training their children in the culture of respecting one another and sharing ideas. (Ka, male)

Mutual respect between the spouses could provide a space to make it easy for them to practically teach the culture of respect to their children.

"Sacrifice" by the Spouses

In traditional marriage life in Rwanda, the spouses could "sacrifice" themselves whenever deemed necessary. They could accept living with their conjugal troubles and stress, in order to protect the well-being of their children. More particularly, the traditional Rwandan woman was steeped in safeguarding the values of Rwandan culture. She could sacrifice her own feelings about her marriage because of the love she had for her children. The rights of her children always prevailed over hers, and such a sacrifice benefited both children and the lastingness of marriage.

A wife would also sacrifice herself for her home; and also for her children even when she had some problems with her husband. She would try to protect her children from any marital difficulties or social shame; she would be patient with her husband's bad behaviour for fear that her children might be the victims of the circumstances. (IN, female)

Women in ancient Rwanda showed their strengths, and also proved that marriage lastingness is possible. When there were problems between the spouses, they would accept sacrificing themselves, i.e., to endure the relationship, in order to protect the well-being of their children. The "sacrifice" by the wife for her household and for her children always led to lastingness of marriage in traditional Rwanda. In unhappy marriages, the children can keep the marriage together (Lauer & Lauer, 1986).

In ancient Rwandan society, the couples had to avoid any decision that could negatively affect the children and victimize them. Marriage was considered an indissoluble institution and divorce was an exceptional event. Rwandan culture recommended polygamy as an alternative to divorce in circumstances of infertility (NISR, 2012). Rwandan culture placed great importance on marriage, and married women and men were given special respect and recognition in society (Uwineza & Pearson, 2009). In cases of trouble within the marriage, divorce was not allowed. The husband would, instead of divorce, go to look for another marriage (NISR, 2012), while the wife was exhorted to be patient under a common traditional saying "*ni ko zubakwa* (that's how marriage is sustained)"!

In the Rwandan traditional marriage life, wives had a central role to play in the well-being of the household. The wives' responsibility included both protecting their children and their marriage. That protection was a priority for them. Instead of the common saying "*iyo amagara atewe hejuru umuntu asama aye*" (when it comes to face a danger [of death], each one first saves his/her life), the wives were generally brave and would sacrifice their own joy and interest. They were always consistent in terms of moral and social responsibilities. They were committed toward the well-being of their children, their husband, their family of origin as well as their family in-law. A wife could accept any type of suffering in whatever she had to do and this was an integral part of her psychosocial responsibilities.

The appreciation of the role played by wives in traditional Rwanda marital life was common. The following are some sayings supporting the above assertion: "*ukurusha umugore akurusha urugo*" ("a man with a better wife has a better household"); "*Umugore ni umutima w'urugo*" ("the wife is the heart of the household"). Conversely, participants in a study complained that Rwandan traditional culture did not value the equality of men and women (Wlodarczyk, 2013). Furthermore, the same study (Wlodarczyk, 2013) suggests the necessity of changes to traditional gender roles in the family and in the society so that equality of men and women can be achieved (Wlodarczyk, 2013). In this sense, the participants make it clear that women, despite being very competent and capable, underestimate their own potential due to lack of self-confidence, and because of having to live under traditional patriarchal values (Wlodarczyk, 2013).

Furthermore, spouses were bonded by cultural values of mutual respect. Misbehaving against the spouse was forbidden in the traditional Rwandan culture. More particularly, a Rwandan husband had the responsibility for taking care of his wife and to avoid making her suffer.

A husband who beat his wife was called an animal. (IN, female)

The spouses had to take care of each other. Mutual devotion and special regard for each other among souses is a factor of marriage lasting-ness (Lauer & Lauer, 1986). Traditional marriages in Africa provided safety and stability (*The New Times*, 2007). Wives' responsibilities in various traditional societies around the world mainly consisted in taking care of their husbands, raising children, responding to domestic needs, and playing related social roles. The husband had to feed and protect the wife and children (Ayisi, 1979). The spouses' failure to fulfill the marital function could lead to family break-up and social shame (Kyalo, 2012). Marriage conferred status and dignity and values. These were fundamentals for the marriage sustainability (Kyalo, 2012).

Spouses' Patience and Perseverance for Marriage as Key Factors for a Strong Household

The concept of patience in marital life expresses the capacity [for the spouses] to accept problems, or suffering without becoming annoyed or anxious (Oxford Dictionaries, 2017). Traditionally, children in Rwanda would listen and obey and go by their parents' advice even in terms of marital life.

> Children would obey their parents…when the problem was becoming complicated; she was told by her mother…"My child: '*ni ko zubakwa*'" [that's how marriage is sustained]…she would obey and know that she had to be patient and cope with difficulties so as to build her household in a strong way. (Ny, female)

In such cases, the wife was guided by her mother and the latter's advice could enable her to cope with any marital problems experienced. She would obey and eventually make a strong household. Participants in this study insisted on the fact that with patience, the spouses who were facing conflicts could easily end up getting on well with each other.

> To be a bit patient could help spouses get on well in the future of their life together. Thanks to perseverance and patience, the couple could realize that disputation was worthless…and after a while the time would come for them to reach a common understanding and settlement of issues. (IN, male)

Patience is among the key features of everyday human experience that have typically been neglected or ignored in mainstream psychological discourse (Kunz, 2002). Patience is the quality of being patient, as the bearing of provocation, annoyance, misfortune, or pain, without complaint, loss of temper, irritation, or the like (Dictionary.com, 1995). There are a number of factors which have been shown as related to long-term marriage. These factors include among others: attitudes towards marital relations (Timothy-Springer & Johnson, 2016); religion (Jeffries, 2006; Mackey & O'Brien, 2005; Mullins, 2016); the role of children (Bachand & Caron, 2001); love, commitment, and intimacy (Phillips et al., 2012); gender (Elliott & Umberson, 2008); communication and conflict resolution (Koraei et al., 2017); support (Landis et al., 2013); attachment and loyalty (Tilse, 1994); and role sharing (Pnina, 2009). Impatient individuals are more likely to experience divorce (De Paola & Gioia, 2017).

Currently, there is not much encouragement in Rwanda for spouses to have patience with their marital lives, which used to be such an important traditional cultural value. This may be caused by modern values that emphasize human rights protection of the spouses. Unfortunately, however, there is a trend to forget that building and living in a good household is also an aspect of human rights. The challenge for today is to find the space to accommodate both aspects, i.e., protecting the spouses against intimate partner violence (Mukashema, 2018) and promoting the marriage lastingness through the respect of traditions in marriage. This should pass through innovative educative strategies for marriage preparation. The elders' views about what they call the patience of wives in traditional marital life in Rwanda pushes one's interrogation of the sense of "*Niko zubakwa*" as traditional advice to a wife facing marital problems (Mukashema, 2018) and what is qualified as intimate partner violence today (Mukashema, 2018).

Is the "*Niko zubakwa*" that was especially spoken to wives, a bad or a good piece of advice in the traditional Rwandan marriage life? Of course, each answer, calling it bad or good, has its own advantages and challenges for marital life. The Rwandan saying of "*Ukurusha umugore akurusha urugo*" (Ny, female) could work also in the situation of sacrifice of the wife for her household.

Marital Life in Rwanda: Traditional Values Versus Modernity

Today, there is a loss of traditional values in marriage life. The loss of these traditional values in married life has a negative impact on marriage lastingness. Marital lastingness was supported by the spouses' families and by the Rwandan culture. Nowadays, traditional practices are under-valued and marriage is becoming more a matter of personal choice of the people involved.

> Even when something significant had happened, because they [spouses] could persevere [in marital life] in the past, the time would come and they would end up having a common understanding and getting on well…- Today spouses do not see any reason as to why one should be patient [in marital life]. (IN, male)

Over time, the dissolution of unions through divorce or death has intensified (NISR, 2012). This situation threatening the marriage and the family is common in the world. The family is concerned by the moral and cultural decline that the world is presently experiencing (Singer, 2019). Today, it is a matter of urgency to bring in the traditional values that were protecting marriages and were ensuring its lastingness.

> We need to pick up some values from those which ancient families were built on, and find a way of relating them to today's situations [of marital life]. We may teach those values to our children because, some of them like patience…even though they might not be practiced as our parents and grandparents did at their time, are missing. (REAF, female)

Participants in this research deplored the fact that some values on which family life was built in traditional Rwanda are lost. They suggest that there is a dire need to go back to the culture and bring in those values. This includes among other factors, patience in marital life, which traditionally supported marriage lastingness and the psychosocial well-being of the household and the families' members. Today's institution of marriage has degenerated, because of the many challenges it faces (Kyalo, 2012). However, it should be noted that Rwandan traditional culture and society have much to teach, and it is never too late to regain and restore the traditional consistency of the institution of marriage, and especially to consider their customs in solving today's marital problems (Ndushabandi et al., 2016). There are relevant and useful values in African spirituality to enrich marriage today (Kyalo, 2012).

To find a solution to this situation in which the family is suffering and even broken-up, threatening the family members' health (MIGE-PROF, 2011; Mukashema, 2014; Mukashema & Sapsofod, 2013), it is imperative to reconcile two realities. On the one hand, there is a need to consider the place and the role of women in traditional Rwandan society such as "a man with a better wife has a better household" and "the wife is the heart of the household." On the other hand, it is also crucial to support women that still keep underestimating their own potential, because of lack of self-confidence as a result of the traditional patriarchal values (Wlodarczyk, 2013). Therefore, the solution to this dilemma should first of all aim to enable wives to estimate and express their own potential. Building on that, the same wives should be encouraged to keep their traditional psychosocial responsibility of protecting marriage to prevent its destruction, an alarming situation being witnessed today (MIGEPROF, 2011; Mukashema, 2014; Mukashema & Sapsford, 2013).

The Idea of Today's "Too Much Freedom" in Spouses

From the experience of the participants in the focus group discussions, it is understood that spouses in post-genocide Rwandan society have too much freedom when compared to the situation in pre-genocide Rwandan society.

A difference between marital homes in ancient Rwandan society and those of Rwandan society today is that today there is too much freedom compared to the customary Rwandan time. In the latter, there were cultural safeguards which provided that spouses could avoid falling into situations of shame, and there was also marital secrecy as a value. There was secrecy and avoidance of disappointment. One would avoid being the object of disappointment of his extended families of origin. Today, there is no place for the family, the spouses are individualistic. (IN, male)

Conclusion

Marriage in traditional Rwanda was protected by a number of psychosocial and cultural values. These included mutual respect, patience, and perseverance, which were seen as key to marriage lastingness. There was psychosocial consideration of the two spouses' respective families of origin in their new household life. The spouses had an exceptionally high-level commitment to marriage life sustainability, because each spouse wanted to avoid being the cause of marriage destruction, or the breakdown of the ties built between their two families, and thus the shame to the families. Therefore, the traditional Rwandan spouses had a psychological feeling of protecting, not only their marriage, but also the ties established between their two families of origin. Currently, there is a loss of traditional cultural values that can upgrade marriage lastingness that were observed in the past.

Participants in this study expressed the need for a recovery of some traditional values in marriage which could prevent today's alarming epidemic of marriage suffering and destruction. To find a solution to the today's situation of marital and family suffering, it is important to accept that culture and society have a lot to teach and it is never too late to regain and restore the traditional consistency of the institution of marriage and family. There are relevant and useful values in African spirituality to enrich marriage today (Kyalo, 2012).

The husband should recover his sense of responsibility for being the protector of the household, i.e., of the marriage and the family. It is imperative to reconcile two realities. On the one hand, there is a need to consider the place and the role of women in the ancient Rwandan society such as "a man with a better wife has a better household" and "the wife is the heart of the household" as has been quoted above. On the other hand, it is crucial to support women that still keep underestimating their own potential because of lack of self-confidence as a result of the traditional patriarchal values (Wlodarczyk, 2013). Therefore, the solution to this dilemma should first of all aim to enable wives to estimate and express their own potential. Once this happens, the same wives should be encouraged to keep their psychosocial responsibility for protecting marriage in preventing its destruction, as was the situation in pre-genocide Rwandan society.

The findings from this research will be of interest for policymakers, mental health and psychosocial support providers, researchers into marriage and the family, etc. Even if data from focus group discussions may not be generalized, the cultural context of the current findings allow for an extendable insight into how marital life in the traditional Rwandan society was lived, and some experiences can be taken from there, built on, and adapted for home-grown solutions for a better and healthier marital life in today's Rwandan society. Drawing from some of the ancestors' customs in marriage life, and adapting them properly to today's marital life conditions, would be of benefit to the marriage institution both at the present time and also in the days to come. Spouses in contemporary Rwanda can learn a lot from their ancestors in ancient Rwanda. Further research on what behaviors may be taken from the Rwandan past can be of interest.

Acknowledgements This research was conducted through the financial support of the University of Rwanda-Sweden Program.

Early Version Presentation
Some aspects of the content of this chapter were presented at the Rome International Conference on Research in Social Science & Humanities (ICRSSH), April 30–May 1, 2019 and published in its linked journal "PEOPLE: International Journal of Social Sciences." Unfortunately, later on, it was found that "grds publishing," the journal's publisher, is listed as a predatory publisher.

Declaration of Interest Statement
There is no conflict of interest.

References

Ayisi, E. O. (1979). *An introduction to the study of African culture* (2nd ed.). Heinemann Educational.

Bachand, L. L., & Caron, S. L. (2001). Ties that bind: A qualitative study of happy long-term marriages. *Contemporary Family Therapy, 23*(1), 105–121. https://doi.org/10.1023/a:1007828317271.

De Paola, M., & Gioia, F. (2017). Does patience matter in marriage stability? Some evidence from Italy. *Review of Economics of the Household, 15*(2), 549–577. https://doi.org/10.1007/s11150-014-9275-4.

Dictionary.com. (1995). *Definition of patience*. https://www.dictionary.com/bro wse/patience.

Elliott, S., & Umberson, D. (2008). The performance of desire: Gender and sexual negotiation in long-term marriages. *Journal of Marriage and the Family, 70*(2), 391–406. https://doi.org/10.1111/j.1741-3737.2008.004 89.x.

Jeffries, V. (2006). Religiosity, benevolent love, and long-lasting marriages. *Humboldt Journal of Social Relations, 30*(1), 77–106. https://www.jstor.org/stable/23263207.

Karimi, R., Bakhtiyari, M., & Arani, A. M. (2019). Protective factors of marital stability in long-term marriage globally: A systematic review. *Epidemiology and Health, 41,*. https://doi.org/10.4178/epih.e2019023.

Koraei, A., Mehr, R. K., Sodani, M., & Aslani, K. (2017). Identification of the factors contributing to satisfying stable marriages in women. *Journal of Family Counseling & Psychotherapy, 6,* 129–164.

Kunz, G. (2002). Simplicity, humility, patience. In E. E. Gantt & R. N. Williams (Eds.), *Psychology for the other: Levinas, ethics and the practice of psychology* (pp. 118–142). Duquesne University Press.

Kyalo, P. (2012, April). A reflection on the African traditional values of marriage and sexuality. *International Journal of Academic Research in Progressive Education and Development, 1*(2). https://pdf4pro.com/amp/view/a-ref lection-on-the-africantraditional-values-of-marriage-58697c.html.

Landis, M., Peter-Wight, M., Martin, M., & Bodenmann, G. (2013). Dyadic coping and marital satisfaction of older spouses in long-term marriage. *GeroPsych: The Journal of Gerontopsychology and Geriatric Psychiatry, 26*(1), 39–47. https://doi.org/10.1024/1662-9647/a000077.

Lauer, R. H., & Lauer, J, C. (1986). Factors in long-term marriages. *Journal of Family Issues, 7*(4), 382–390. https://doi.org/10.1177/019251386007 004003.

Le, B., & Agnew, C. R. (2003). Commitment and its theorized determinants: A meta-analysis of the investment model. *Personal Relationships, 10,* 37–57. https://doi.org/10.1111/1475-6811.00035.

Mackey, R. A., & O'Brien, B. A. (2005). The significance of religion in lasting marriages. *Journal of Religion, Spirituality & Aging, 1,* 35–63. https://doi.org/10.1300/j496v18n01_04.

MIGEPROF [Ministry of Gender and Family Promotion]. (2011). *National policy on fighting against gender-based violence*. Kigali. https://migeprof.gov.rw/fileadmin/_migrated/content_uploads/GBV_Policy-2_1_.pdf.

Mukashema, I. (2014). Facing domestic violence for mental health in Rwanda: Opportunities and challenges. *Procedia-Social and Behavioral Sciences, 591–598*. https://doi.org/10.1016/j.sbspro.2014.04.476.

Mukashema, I. (2018). A report about intimate partner violence in southern and western Rwanda. *International Journal of Child, Youth and Family Studies, 9*(3), 68–99. https://doi.org/10.18357/ijcyfs93201818277.

Mukashema, I., & Sapsford, R. (2013). Marital conflicts in Rwanda: Points of view of Rwandan psycho-socio-medical professionals. *Procedia-Social and Behavioral Sciences, 82*(2013), 149–168. https://doi.org/10.1016/j.sbspro.2013.06.239.

Mullins, D. (2016). The effects of religion on enduring marriages. *Social Sciences, 5*, 24. https://doi.org/10.3390/socsci5020024.

Ndushabandi, E. N., Kagaba, M., & Gasafari, W. (2016). *Intra-family conflicts in Rwanda: A constant challenge to sustainable peace in Rwanda*. http://www.irdp.rw/wp-content/uploads/2019/02/intrafamily-conflicts-last-version-2.pdf.

NISR [National Institute of Statistics Rwanda], Ministry of Finance and Economic Planning, Ministry of Health and ICF International. (2012, February). *Demographic and health survey 2010*. NISR, MOH and ICF International. https://dhsprogram.com/pubs/pdf/FR259/FR259.pdf.

Oxford Dictionaries. (2017). *Definition of patience in English by Oxford dictionaries*. Oxford University Press. https://en.oxforddictionaries.com/definition/patience.

Phillips, T. M., Wilmoth, J. D., & Marks, L. D. (2012). Challenges and conflicts…strengths and supports: A study of enduring African American marriages. *Journal of Black Studies 43*(8), 936–952. https://doi.org/10.1177/0021934712463237.

Pnina, R. (2009). The differences in role division between partners in long-term marriages and their well-being. *Journal of Family Social Work, 12*, 44–55. https://doi.org/10.1080/10522150802667106.

Quinn, N. (1996). Culture and contradiction: The case of Americans reasoning marriage. *Ethos: Journal of the Society for Psychological Anthropology, 24*(3), 391–425. https://doi.org/10.1525/eth.1996.24.3.02a00010.

Quinn, N. (2019). American marriage revisited in the light of human evolution. *Ethos, 47*(3), 263–280. https://doi.org/10.1111/etho.12246.

Schoebi, D., Karney, B. R., & Bradbury, T. N. (2012). Stability and change in the first 10 years of marriage: does commitment confer benefits beyond the effects of satisfaction? *Journal of Personality and Social Psychology, 102*(4), 729–742. https://doi.org/10.1037/a0026290.

Singer, P. (2019). *Beyond the traditional family.* https://www.newtimes.co.rw/opinions/beyond-traditional-family.

Stanley, S. M., Rhoades, G. K., & Whitton, S. W. (2010). Commitment: Functions, formation, and the securing of romantic attachment. *Journal of Family Theory & Review, 2*, 243–257. https://doi.org/10.1111/j.1756-2589.2010.00060.x.

Swensen, C. H., & Trahaug, G. (1985). Commitment and the long-term marriage relationship. *Journal of Marriage and Family, 47*(4), 939–945. https://www.jstor.org/stable/352337.

The New Times. (2007, October 13). Is traditional marriage still valid? https://www.newtimes.co.rw/section/read/85869.

Thompson, C. (2017, June 27). *Marriage in Africa.* https://www.birmingham.ac.uk/schools/historycultures/research/news/2017/marriage-in-africa.aspx.

Tilse, C. (1994). Long term marriage and long term care "we thought we'd be together till we died". *Australasian Journal on Ageing 13*(4), 172–174. https://doi.org/10.1111/j.1741-6612.1994.tb00666.x.

Timothy-Springer, R., & Johnson, E. J. (2016). Qualitative study on the experiences of married couples. *Journal of Human Behavior in the Social Environment, 28*(7), 889–902. https://doi.org/10.1080/10911359.2018.1467291.

Tzitzika, M., Lampridis, E., & Kalamaras, D. (2020). Relational satisfaction of spousal/partner informal caregivers of people with multiple sclerosis: Relational commitment, caregiving burden, and prorelational behavioral tendencies. *International Journal of MS Care, 22*(2), 60–66. https://doi.org/10.7224/1537-2073.2019-003.

Uwineza, P., & Pearson, E. (2009). *Sustaining women's gains in Rwanda: The influence of indigenous culture and post-genocide politics.* Hunt Alternatives Fund. https://www.inclusivesecurity.org/wp-content/uploads/2012/08/1923_sustaining_womens_gains_nocover.pdf.

Wlodarczyk, K. (2013). *Doing gender, doing leadership. A phenomenological study of women in leadership positions in Kigali, Rwanda.* Lund University library. http://lup.lub.lu.se/luur/download?func=downloadFile&recordOId=3798889&fileOId=3798932.

7

Prevention and Management of Destructive Marital Conflict in Pre-genocide Rwandan Society

Immaculée Mukashema, Joseph Gumira Hahirwa, Alexandre Hakizamungu, and Lambert Havugintwari

Introduction

Marriage and health are found to be closely related (Kiecolt-Glaser & Newton, 2001; Robles et al., 2014; Whisman & Baucom, 2011). Being married is associated with better health (Kiecolt-Glaser & Newton, 2001). Marriage seems to be an advantage to the mental health of married people (Fincham, 2003). However, the health impact of marriage is affected by marital quality (Kiecolt-Glaser & Newton, 2001). Marital conflict (Fincham, 2009; Mukashema & Sapsford, 2013) or marital disaccord (Burnet, 2011), marital disagreements, problems, and instability (Johnson et al., 1986), marital happiness and interaction (Johnson et al., 1986) are among the multiple dimensions of marital quality. The dimensions of marital quality vary and can be distinguished into intrapersonal and interpersonal dimensions (Nurhayati et al., 2019).

I. Mukashema (✉) · J. Gumira Hahirwa · A. Hakizamungu ·
L. Havugintwari
College of Arts and Social Sciences, University of Rwanda, Butare, Rwanda

© The Author(s), under exclusive license to Springer Nature
Switzerland AG 2021
I. Mukashema (ed.), *Psychosocial Well-Being and Mental Health of Individuals in Marital and in Family Relationships in Pre- and Post-Genocide Rwanda*,
https://doi.org/10.1007/978-3-030-74560-8_7

Conflict is obvious in marital relations (Argyle & Furnham 1983; Goeke-Morey et al., 2003; McCoy et al., 2009). Marital conflict may be constructive or destructive (Goeke-Morey et al., 2003; McCoy et al., 2009). Marital conflict is said to be constructive when spouses deal with conflict in positive ways by displaying behaviors, such as verbal and physical affection, problem solving and support (Goeke-Morey et al., 2003; McCoy et al., 2009). Constructive conflict tends to be cooperative, pro-social, and relationship-preserving in nature (Deutsch, 1973). Deutsch (1973) argues that constructive behaviors are relatively positive in emotional tone.

Marital conflict is described as destructive when it is hostile, angry, and contains conflict tactics such as physical aggression, verbal aggression, threat, and personal insult (Goeke-Morey et al., 2003; McCoy et al., 2009). Destructive conflict is competitive, antisocial, and relationship-damaging in nature. Deutsch (1973) states that destructive behaviors exhibit negativity, disagreeableness, and sometimes hostility (Deutsch, 1973). To benefit mental health in marital life, marriage should be lived without destructive marital conflict, which is a dimension of marital quality.

As marital conflict is inevitable (Argyle & Furnham, 1983; Goeke-Morey et al., 2003; McCoy et al., 2009), marital conflict can have negative impacts on various aspects. The marital relation itself can be affected such as marital and family disharmony (McCoy et al., 2009), divorce (Amato & Keith, 1991; Emery, 1982). The spouses' health may be impacted (Kiecolt-Glaser & Newton, 2001). Hostile marital conflict has a negative impact on children's self-esteem, achievement in school, and increases the likelihood of depression and antisocial behavior (Gottman, 1979; Jenkins & Smith, 1991; McCoy et al., 2009; Montemayor, 1983). Lloyd (1990) suggests that conflict that is recurrent and stable over time is most problematic for marital relational stability.

There should be mechanisms to prevent or/and to appropriately deal with destructive marital conflict to avoid various negative consequences. Researchers suggest that the inability to constructively manage conflict between spouses themselves is much more important in affecting child adjustment problems than separation and divorce (Amato & Keith, 1991; Emery, 1982). Managing marital conflict and the manner couples manage their conflict has an impact on marital health (Fincham, 2003). Marital conflict resolution is among the factors which determine the impact of the conflict on the relationship (Reese-Weber & Bartle-Haring, 1998).

Marital conflict, family conflict, and domestic violence have recently gained the interest as an area of scientific research in Rwanda. The interest of research in the area of marital conflict, family conflict, and domestic violence is influenced by the increase of conflict among spouses and among parents and children (MIGEPROF, 2011; Mukashema & Sapsford, 2013; Ndushabandi et al., 2016) in post-genocide Rwandan society. Marital conflict in post-genocide Rwandan society is a health issue as such that professionals are being consulted by spouses experiencing that problem (Mukashema & Sapsford, 2013).

The problem of marital conflict has been insufficiently explored in Rwanda (Mukashema & Sapsford, 2013) and only a small number of publications about Rwanda can be found after the genocide of 1994 perpetrated against the Tutsis. The year 1994 is often taken as a reference time separating the pre- and post-periods in relation to the genocide. It is observed that concepts such as marital conflict (Mukashema & Sapsford, 2013) and marital disaccord (Burnet, 2011) are quite newly used in Rwanda (Mukashema, 2014). Little is academically known about psychosocial life in marriage and family in the pre-genocide Rwandan society. Having searched via Rwandan elders with experience in marital life in ancient Rwandan society, the researchers, in this specific chapter, intend to report on the finding regarding the ways which were used to deal with destructive marital conflict in customary Rwanda.

The chapter presents the outcomes from the field data collected during focus group discussions with Rwandan elders. The focus group discussions were held with a mixed group made up of two males and three females selected I from the "Guardian of memory" known as *Inteko Izirikana* (IN) located in Kigali city; a mixed group made up of five males and two females from Rwanda Elders Advisory Forum (RE) in Kigali City; two homogeneous groups made up of seven males and eleven females respectively, selected from the district of Nyanza (Ny) of the southern province of Rwanda; and two homogeneous groups made up of eight males and seven females respectively, selected from the district of

Karongi (Ka) of the western province of Rwanda. The data were collected and analyzed using methodological approaches detailed in Chapter 2 of this volume.

Destructive marital conflict in new households was prevented in ancient Rwandan society. Once destructive marital conflict had risen despite preventive measures in place, social mechanisms were put into action to handle it.

Prevention of Destructive Marital Conflict in New Households in Ancient Rwandan Society

The prevention of destructive marital conflict in new households would mainly and primarily run through the family in the parental life process. The parental marital daily lifestyle played an important role in preventing destructive marital conflict for the future spouses. It was a kind of training based on a family lifestyle aiming at the preparation of young people for their future marriage and for their subsequent marital life. Second, prevention was possible through verbal pieces of advice given to young people just prior to their marriage. The young people always observed their parents while living with them, and were advised not to have fights between themselves at home. They had to seek for help from their parents in cases of misunderstanding.

> The young people used to observe their parents living carefully and peacefully in their own marital life. This would teach them that they would also have to avoid destructive marital conflict when they got married. (REAF, male)

> In their respective family of origin, the bride and the groom were well prepared for their marriage through the observation to their own parents' behaviors. They were told that if ever a controversial thing was to happen to them once married, they should not fight each other. They should

rather approach the parents and tell them what was going wrong. Therefore, the parents could take part in a controversial situation to help them
manage and even solve it. (Ny, female)

The young people were well prepared for the marital life ahead of
marriage time so that their marital life could function well. They were
told that if something was to disrupt their relationship, they shouldn't
fight each other. They would rather have to approach the parents and tell
them about the experienced situation, and then the parents would listen
to them and advise them. (Ny, male)

Within the marital and parental life in ancient Rwandan society, the children used to learn by observing the living behaviors of their parents. The
parents' behaviors were guided by observation of a number of cultural
values which could lead to a peaceful life in the households. The children
used to learn by observing how to live peacefully through mutual respect.
They would observe how their parents were living in harmony. In the
eyes of their children, the parents would avoid bad behaviors that were
against the culture of peace. Parents were expected to live and behave
carefully in an exemplary manner to set an example to their children who
were to become spouses in the future. Once married, the young spouses
had to live carefully and peacefully in their turn, and this was seen as an
important value they had learned from their parents. Thus, this would
prevent destructive marital conflict between them. Through observation,
the children could also learn how each had to fulfill his/her responsibilities as a future spouse. This learning by observation was indirectly one
way of preventing destructive marital conflict in the new households.
Destructive marital conflict prevention was also made possible through
verbal pieces of advice, which specifically were given to the young people
about to get married on what course of action they should take in case
of conflict in the new household.

On the one hand, the young people were advised not to fight each
other. They were instead advised to report any misunderstanding to
their parents and get help from them before it might lead to destructive marital conflict. On the other hand, even if they were encouraged
to search for help from their families in case of misunderstanding, the

new spouses were trained before their marriage to be very careful and to abstain from offending their partner. They would strive not to be blamed by their families because of conflict between them. They were fearful of shame if ever they had had a conflict between them and their families came to know about it.

> Long ago, there was safety and stability in the households in Rwanda because the disputes were resolved by the spouses within their household. This was so because of the fear of the spouses to be blamed due to a conflict. The spouses would fear to commit offenses to one another as this could prompt their parents to blame them. (REAF, male)

Even if the new spouses were exhorted to search for their families' help in cases of conflict, living in destructive conflict was a shame for them in the eyes of their families. Therefore, they were exhorted to avoid conflict, or solve any conflict them by themselves, for fear of being blamed and therefore suffering the shame of the existence of conflict in their household. Failure to do so would prompt the parents to intervene in the spousal conflict to help in managing/solving it. The way couples manage their conflict influences the whole family system (Fincham, 2003).

Spousal Destructive Conflict Management in the Families of Origin

Despite the efforts to prevent destructive marital conflict in the new households, it was possible to experience some conflict situations. In those situations, there were social mechanisms in place to handle them through the spouses' families of origin. The parents of the spouses would help their children to overcome the situation of destructive conflict among them. There was a societal framing spirit used to help the married couples in ancient Rwandan society. A problem arising between the spouses could be resolved within and inside the families; it could not go outside the spouses' families of origin.

Following their marriage, the new spouses would become members of the society made by the two families of origin. These families had a way of doing a "framing" for the married couple. That framing was also meant to take care of the new spouses in helping them manage potential destructive conflicts rising between them. When a petty fault destructive conflict occurred among the spouses, this destructive conflict was handled immediately to avoid the spread of information to the public. (REAF, female)

In some cases of destructive conflict, the wife could decide to go quietly to see either her mother-in-law or her own mother, and would tell them what kind of conflict was happening in her home. After listening to her daughter-in-law/her daughter, the mother-in-law/native mother might find that the wife was wrong herself. In this case, this is what she could tell her: ["My daughter, in hearing what you said, I can see that you have wronged your husband. Please repent on this fault and go back to your home. Be perseverant and patient with your husband. A husband is a chief; he is a chief for his wife and the whole household. You have to be careful toward your husband, go and behave in this and/or in that way"]. She would go on saying, "We will have to see your husband too and we will blame him." Then, the mother-in law could go and exhort her son to stop beating his wife. As a result of this mediation, the wife with her husband would thrive and make their family peaceful. The wife would follow the mother's advice, to go back home and together with her husband, they could prosper and make a good family. (IN, female)

In days of yore, when the spouses quarreled, the parents could come together and listen to the two spouses arguing about their negative conflict. Then, the parents, having understood what the problem was, could tell one of them: ["You (the wife or to the husband) are mistaken]. How come that you fight with your spouse every day while we know well that you got married loving each other? Your disputes will not help your home at all, we have given you a spouse to build up a household, not a wife to quarrel with, go back to your home and do not negatively conflict any more"]. In the past, there was a common understanding in such a way when the elders had warned the new spouses. The latter would eventually listen and comply with what the elders had given as advice. Such advice was to be valued. (Ka, female)

Even with marital conflict prevention, marital conflict is a common aspect of marital relations (Delatorre & Wagner, 2018; Theiss & Leustek, 2016). When a destructive conflict occurred among the new spouses, they would by themselves or with the help of the parents, handle it immediately so as not to let the information spread to the public. Whenever the parents had warned someone among the new spouses, there was a common understanding of the situation. He/she would internalize what the parents had given as advice and the advice was respected as such. The conflict management is key to a successful marriage (Fincham, 2003). African traditional mechanisms of conflict prevention, management, and resolution were largely effective and respected. The decisions about the conflict were binding to all concerned parties. This was mostly because the identity of individual spouse was linked to that of his or her family and the two families were formed by the acceptance of marriage alliances (Ademowo, 2015).

In the ancient Rwandan society, the new spouses would become members of the large community made up of the two families. These families would have a way of doing a framing for the married couple. That framing would ensure that the new spouses were taken care of, by helping them to manage destructive conflict arising between them. Both the parents-in-law as well as the parents of origin had an important role to play in destructive marital conflict management for their married children. This was done in order to prevent their children divorcing, and therefore the breaking down of the relationships established between their two families through the marriage of their two children. Thanks to the involvement of the families of origin in social framing in marriage, in destructive marital conflict prevention and management, the ancient households were stable and long lasting.

The wife would play a great role in maintaining the marital relationship in the ancient Rwandan society. She was encouraged to be patient and persevering in remaining at her home, even when she was a victim of destructive conflicts with her husband. These encouragements from the parents were typically voiced as common sayings from the mother or the mother-in-law as follows: "My daughter, please stay there at your home; that is how the families are made up." The husband was also reminded of his responsibilities; e.g., that he had to care about his wife and especially to avoid destructive conflict with her. The call upon the wife to patience and perseverance, was accompanied by blaming and advising the husband about his responsibility to respect his wife, and getting rid of destructive behavior such as beating her.

"Kwahukana"

The *Kwahukana* phenomenon [to flee the marital home for a relatively short period]: sometimes a spouse (generally the wife) could flee the marital home in a situation of conflict. She could flee from her husband for a relatively short period of time (*kwahukana*). She would go to her in-law family or to her family of origin. Thereafter, the management of the conflict could be initiated within the family to where the wife had fled.

> When the two spouses had failed to resolve the conflict between them, the wife could flee to her family of origin or to her family in-law. After one or two days, the husband could come to the family where his wife was to get her back home. The husband would be asked to explain what he had done to his wife to such an extent that she ended up leaving their home. It was such a long discussion indeed. After listening to both parties, the parents would deliberate and the blame would go to the wrongdoer. Eventually, they could advise the two spouses to go back home and live in a peaceful way. (Ny, female)

> In some cases of conflict between the spouses, the wife could flee to her family of origin. Then later, the husband would come to her family of origin and try to get her back home. There was a deliberation about the conflict and sometimes agreement was not reached. In this case, the wife's family of origin could call upon the family-in-law for further deliberations. The two families would gather to reconcile the spouses in conflict. They would carefully listen to what the real matter was in order to devise a way forward. The parents would blame one or both of the couple, following the allegations leveled against each of them. The parents would then teach the spouses what they should do in order to live in peace and to build a strong household. The reconciled spouses thereafter had

to go back home, ensure that they respected each other, and they would eventually live a prosperous marital life for the rest of their lives. (Ny, male)

The wife could flee her husband and go to live in her family of origin. Her husband would go and try to get her back home. There was what can be called a "socio-family court" made up of both families to settle the matter. Each spouse would defend him/herself, depending on allegations leveled against them. The parents would listen to them and help them to resolve the conflict. They would then request the spouses to go back home and live in peace. (IN, male)

In situation of spousal destructive conflict, the wife could either flee her husband to her native family, or go to her family-in-law. The boy's family would often defend their daughter-in-law. I never saw my sister-in-law fleeing to her father's family whenever there were marital problems. She would always flee from her husband to her father-in-law. This situation was not even revealed to her father's family. Everything was handled so secretly. Then her father-in-law could take her to her husband's home to reconcile the couple. In ancient Rwandan society, the parents had this kind of power over their children. When the wife was a victim of marital disputes, her family-in-law had to protect her. (RE, male)

"*Kwahukana*," i.e., a woman feeling fed up with her husband's treatment and then deciding to leave her home, was seen as a special event in the course of spousal conflict resolution. Fleeing either to the family-in-law or to her family of origin by the wife would give her a safe and secure sanctuary. The fleeing spouse (generally the wife) who was previously in danger, would now have protection and feel safe. The other spouse (generally the husband) had to stay at home alone, take time to think about the situation, and then decide to go to try to bring his wife back. The separation time was a good opportunity for them to take time to reflect on their conflict, receive advice from their families, and to refresh their marital relations and life together. Likewise, this thinking-time would also enable them to drop their conflict and decide to continue their marital journey peacefully.

The role of the families in managing and ensuring good marital relationships of their married children in ancient Rwandan society was consistent with the general African traditional families. These families played important roles in supporting the new spouses' good marital relations (Chereji & King, 2015). In ancient Rwandan society, the two families of origin were actively involved in the new household's destructive marital conflict management. This was so important in order the help the new spouses get on well, but also to maintain the link and the unity established between the two families through the marriage of the two young people. It was people's conviction that even though a married couple was made up of two persons, both their families also felt bound by those two young person's marriage. All was put into play to maintain the new spouses in living together in a peaceful way. Preventing new destructive spousal conflict and intervening in the management of arising conflict would be everyone's concern in the ancient Rwandan society, and the aim was to safeguard marriage.

Preventing and managing destructive marital conflict in traditional African societies—including Rwanda—was largely about the prevention of divorce as a potential consequence of destructive marital conflict. Divorce was viewed as a shameful situation (Chereji & King, 2015). The parents would do everything they could to prevent divorce. The voices of parents as elders was always listened to, since they had a measure of power over their children and were respected by them. This was common to traditional African cultures which acknowledged the elders as the guardians of the secrets of life, and as the "the wise ones" to be obeyed in the prevention of conflict, and for the preservation of peace (Stuckelberger, 2005).

In ancient Rwandan society, the new spouses were aware of the fact that they were living in their own household, but also within a wider community made up especially of their two families of origin. They knew very well that the community members around them were always looking at them. In that context, the spouses would resolve the destructive marital conflict between them as soon as it arose, so that it could not become publicaly known. In the latter scenario, this would bring shame upon them. However, in cases where they had failed to hide their conflict, their parents were ready to fully listen to them and to help them recover their normal course of peaceful marital life. Destructive conflict among the new spouses was a shameful situation for the two families of origin. Therefore, these families would contribute to the prevention and the management of such a situation in order to maintain the spouses in the marital relation and thus safeguarding the link between two families established as a result of the marriage of their two young people. Commonly in African traditional societies, there was thus an important role for families in marriage conflict management and resolution (Waindim, 2018).

Conclusion

In ancient Rwandan society, there were cultural ways of preventing, managing, and resolving destructive marital conflict in new households. Destructive marital conflict was prevented thanks to the training that the children could get through the marital lifestyle of their parents. Prevention was also possible through verbal advice that prospective spouses would get prior to their marriage. Whenever the conflict occurred despite constant efforts to prevent it, it was first managed within the new household. In case this had failed to function at this level, the two families would help the spouses resolve the conflict so as to allow the marital life to continue in a peaceful manner. The two spouses' families of origin were crucial in the new destructive spousal marital conflict management and resolution, whenever the conflict could not be solved by the spouses themselves. The families would abide by the principle of objectivity while helping the spouses get through the destructive conflict. In cases of a destructive conflict, the wife could flee the marital home to her family-in-law or to her family of origin. It would normally take some days before the husband would try to get his wife back. The husband would only succeed in getting his wife back home after he had had discussions with the family to where she had fled, and sometimes in the presence of the two families together. Such discussions were focused on the reasons that had led to the conflict in question. Deliberations would always end in blaming the wrongdoer in this.

The spouses were then told to go back to their home and continue their marital journey. There were various ways the two families could contribute to the prevention and management of the destructive marital conflict in the new household; and for a number of reasons. The two families could advise the wives to have patience and perseverance, or blame the husbands for the wrong done. The reasons behind these efforts included the prevention of divorce, making the new household last a long time, and maintaining the ties established between the two families. Both families were supportive to the new spouses in cases of marital conflict to such an extent that the family-in-law of the married woman could even protect and defend her.

This chapter provides an academic reference for marital conflict prevention and management within the customary Rwandan society available to the academic readership. It describes the Rwandan-/African-society methods which were used to prevent and to deal with marital conflict and domestic violence. These ways can also be of inspiration today, in finding solutions to situations of destructive marital conflict within Rwandan society. The findings presented in the chapter will be of interest for, among others: policymakers, mental health and psychosocial support providers, and researchers into marriage and the family. Even if data from focus group discussions may not be eligible for generalization, the cultural context of the current findings give an insight into how marital life within traditional Rwandan society was organized, regarding the prevention and handling of marital conflict. Some experiences can be used from these earlier customs, can be built on, and adapted to home-grown solutions for a better and healthier marital life in today's Rwandan society. However, a further extended research covering the whole Rwandan country could be of considerable interest. It could systematically look at the dimensions of marital quality in Rwandan society at large today.

Acknowledgements This research was conducted through the financial support of the University of Rwanda-Sweden Program.

Declaration of Interest Statement
There is no conflict of interest.

References

Ademowo, A. J. (2015). *Conflict management in traditional African society.* https://www.researchgate.net/publication/281749510.

Amato, P. R., & Keith, B. (1991). Parental divorce and the well-being of children: A meta-analysis. *Psychological Bulletin, 110,* 26–46. https://doi.org/10.1037/0033-2909.110.1.26.

Argyle, M., & Furnham, A. (1983). Sources of satisfaction and conflict in long-term relationships. *Journal of Marriage and the Family, 45*(3), 481–493. https://doi.org/10.2307/351654.

Burnet, J. E. (2011). Women have found respect: Gender quotas, symbolic representation, and female empowerment in Rwanda. *Politics & Gender, 7,* 303–334. https://doi.org/10.1017/S1743923X11000250.

Chereji, C.-R., & King, C. W. (2015). Aspects of traditional conflict management practices among the Ogoni of Nigeria. *Conflict Studies Quarterly, 10,* 56–68.

Delatorre, M. Z., & Wagner, A. (2018). Marital conflict management of married men and women. *Psico-USF, 23*(2). https://doi.org/10.1590/1413-82712018230204.

Deutsch, M. (1973). *The Resolution of Conflict: Constructive and Destructive Processes.* New Haven, CT: Yale University Press.

Emery, R. E. (1982). Interparental conflict and the children of discord and divorce. *Psychological Bulletin, 92*(2), 310–330. https://doi.org/10.1037/0033-2909.92.2.310.

Fincham, F. D. (2003). Marital conflict: Correlates, structure and context. *Current Directions in Psychological Science, 12*(23), 23–27. https://doi.org/10.1111/1467-8721.01215.

Fincham, F. D. (2009). *Marital happiness: The encyclopedia of positive psychology.* Blackwell.

Goeke-Morey, M. C., Cummings, E. M., Harold, G. T., & Shelton, K. H. (2003). Categories and continua of destructive and constructive marital conflict tactics from the perspective of U.S. and Welsh children. *Journal of Family Psychology, 17*(3), 327–338. https://doi.org/10.1037/0893-3200.17.3.327.

Gottman, J. M. (1979). *Marital interaction: Experimental investigations.* Academic Press.

Jenkins, J. M., & Smith, M. A. (1991). Marital disharmony and children's behavior problems: Aspects of a poor marriage that affect children adversely.

Journal of Child Psychology and Psychiatry and Allied Disciplines, 32, 793–810.

Johnson, D. R., White, L. K., Edwards, J. N., & Booth, A. (1986). Dimensions of marital quality: Toward methodological and conceptual refinement. *Journal of Family Issues, 7*(1), 31–49. https://doi.org/10.1177/019251386007001003.

Kiecolt-Glaser, J. K., & Newton, T. L. (2001). Marriage and health: *His and Hers. Psychological Bulletin, 127*(4), 472–503. https://doi.org/10.1037/0033-2909.127.4.472.

Lloyd, S. A. (1990). A behavioral self-report technique for assessing conflict in close relationships. *Journal of Social and Personal Relationships, 7*(2), 265–272. https://doi.org/10.1177/0265407590072007.

McCoy, K., Cummings, E. M., & Davies, P. T. (2009). Constructive and destructive marital conflict, emotional security and children's prosocial behavior. *Journal of Child Psychology and Psychiatry, 50*(3), 270–279. https://doi.org/10.1111/j.1469-7610.2008.01945.x.

MIGEPROF [Ministry of Gender and Family Promotion]. (2011). *National policy on fighting against gender-based violence.* Kigali. https://migeprof.gov.rw/fileadmin/_migrated/content_uploads/GBV_Policy-2_1_.pdf.

Montemayor, R. (1983). Parents and adolescents in conflict: All families some of the time and some families most of the time. *The Journal of Early Adolescence, 3*(1–2), 83–103. https://doi.org/10.1177/027243168331007.

Mukashema, I. (2014). Facing domestic violence for mental health in Rwanda: Opportunities and challenges. *Procedia-Social and Behavioral Sciences,* 591–598. https://doi.org/10.1016/j.sbspro.2014.04.476.

Mukashema, I., & Sapsford, R. (2013). Marital conflicts in Rwanda: Points of view of Rwandan psycho-socio-medical professionals. *Procedia-Social and Behavioral Sciences, 82*(2013), 149–168. https://doi.org/10.1016/j.sbspro.2013.06.239.

Ndushabandi, E. N., Kagaba, M., & Gasafari, W. (2016). *Intra-family conflicts in Rwanda: A constant challenge to sustainable peace in Rwanda.* http://www.irdp.rw/wp-content/uploads/2019/02/intrafamily-conflicts-last-version-2.pdf.

Nurhayati, S. R., Faturochman, F., & Helmi, A. K. (2019). Marital quality: A conceptual review. *Buletin Psikologi, 27*(2), 109–124. https://doi.org/10.22146/buletinpsikologi.37691.

Reese-Weber, M., & Bartle-Haring, S. (1998). Conflict resolution styles in family subsystems and adolescent romantic relationships. *Journal of Youth and Adolescence, 27*(6), 735–752. https://doi.org/10.1023/A:102286183 2406.

Robles, T. F., Slatcher, R. B., Trombello, J. M., & McGinn, M. M. (2014). Marital quality and health: A meta-analytic review. *Psychological Bulletin, 140*(1), 140–187. https://doi.org/10.1037/a0031859.

Stuckelberger, A. (2005). *A transgenerational perspective on peace and on violence prevention roles of older persons and grand-parents in the culture and development of peace and non-violence.* Kluwer Edition.

Theiss, J. A., & Leustek, J. (2016). Marital conflict. In C. Shehan (Ed.), *Encyclopedia of family studies* (pp. 1–4). Wiley- Blackwell. https://doi.org/10.1002/9781119085621.wbefs378.

Waindim, J. N. (2018). Traditional methods of conflict resolution: The Kom experience. *Conflict Trends, 4,* 38–44.

Whisman, M. A., & Baucom, D. H. (2011). Intimate relationships and psychopathology. *Clinical Child and Family Psychology Review, 15*(1), 4–13. https://doi.org/10.1007/s10567-011-0107-2.

8

Intimate Partner Violence, Destructive Marital Conflict, Domestic and Family Violence in Post-genocide Rwandan Society

Immaculée Mukashema

Introduction

Intimate partner violence (IPV), also referred to as domestic violence (DV), denotes abusive behavior by either partner or both partners in intimate relationship (Shipway, 2004). Like child abuse and elder abuse, intimate partner violence is a component of domestic and family violence (DFV). Each of these concepts, i.e., intimate partner violence, child abuse, and elder abuse, mean abusive behaviors in which one individual gains power over another individual (Huecker & Smock, 2020).

Intimate partner violence (IPV) refers to any behavior, within intimate relationships, that causes physical, psychological, or sexual harm (WHO, 2012). Intimate partner violence (IPV) or domestic violence (DV) refers to a pattern of threatening, controlling, coercive behavior, violence or abuse (financial, physical, psychological/emotional, and sexual) used by adults or adolescents against their current or former intimate partners

I. Mukashema (✉)
College of Arts and Social Sciences, University of Rwanda, Butare, Rwanda

© The Author(s), under exclusive license to Springer Nature Switzerland AG 2021
I. Mukashema (ed.), *Psychosocial Well-Being and Mental Health of Individuals in Marital and in Family Relationships in Pre- and Post-Genocide Rwanda*, https://doi.org/10.1007/978-3-030-74560-8_8

(Doyle & McWilliams, 2018). IPV violates the fundamental rights of its victims, and has been identified as a public health problem present in all societies (García-Moreno et al., 2013; Krug et al., 2002).

Intimate partner violence (IPV) is a leading public health problem (Izugbara et al., 2020; Shamu et al., 2011). There is a link between poor mental health and IPV and this needs to be considered in healthcare policies and provision (Doyle & McWilliams, 2018). IPV is increasingly recognized as a major public health problem associated with a wide range of serious physical and psychological effects for victims of IPV and their children (World Health Organization [WHO], 2012). IPV is a major source of mental disturbance and psychosocial dysfunction in survivor women (Rees et al., 2016). Physical, sexual, and emotional intimate partner violence cause serious health problems for women (Campbell, 2002).

IPV is a pervasive and devastating health and social problem that affects every population category in all nations (Bragg, 2003). Some cases end in the death of the victim by murder or suicide (Futures Without Violence, 2012; García-Moreno et al., 2013). IPV distresses families and communities. It drains household resources, strains family ties, and depresses family members (Ellsberg et al., 2008). The gravity of IPV's effects are recognized in the latest version of the Diagnostic and Statistical Manual of Mental Disorders, DSM-5, which recognizes marital conflict with violence as a new relational disorder, and thus identifies this behavior as pathological (American Psychiatric Association, 2013).

Some of the existing studies that provide information about the conditions associated with IPV in Rwanda focus on violence against women, connecting it specifically to HIV infection among women (e.g., Kayibanda et al., 2012). Among other studies, Thomson et al. (2015), in examining the factors associated with physical or sexual IPV in Rwanda between 2005 and 2010, noted that in addition to the already occurring IPV-focused initiatives in the health and legal sectors, campaigns are needed to shift public perceptions towards deterrence; that is, towards ending IPV. These deterrence-focused campaigns are especially necessary given Umubyeyi et al. (2016) finding that even if legislative measures have been instituted to protect women from abuse, many Rwandan women do not benefit from those efforts.

Additional studies investigated IPV specific to pregnant women in Rwanda (e.g., Ntaganira et al., 2008) and IPV toward women and its relationship to the mental health of victims and perpetrators (Verduin et al. 2012), while still others focused on the perspectives on IPV and marital conflict of psychologists, social workers, and medical professionals (see, e.g., Mukashema & Sapsford, 2013). Despite the ongoing investigations of IPV, scholarly reports that provide an overview of IPV, marital conflict, domestic and family conflict in Rwanda are few.

Intimate Partner Violence in Post-conflict Societies

While conflict and post-conflict societies in sub-Saharan Africa have a high number under recognized problems of intimate partner violence, there has been limited data on IPV from conflict-affected sub-Saharan African societies (Kinyanda et al., 2016). Although intimate partner violence (IPV) is said to be globally understudied in Africa as a public health problem (Izugbara et al., 2020), some studies of IPV in post-conflict African societies such as in Liberia (Kelly et al., 2018), in Uganda, in Cote D'Ivoire and Liberia (Saile et al., 2013) have been conducted. The research conducted in Liberia (Kelly et al., 2018) has shown that residing in a post-conflict region was associated with post-conflict IPV. The study conducted in Uganda, Cote D'Ivoire, and Liberia (Saile et al., 2013) has found that women who have higher levels of conflict-related abuses also report higher levels of IPV victimization during and after conflict (Saile et al., 2013). It has been noted that post-conflict societies experience globally high rates of domestic and family violence (DFV) committed against women and children (Bradley, 2018). Exposure to political violence and to human rights abuses at the individual level has been linked to higher rates of IPV perpetration among men in conflict and post-conflict settings (Gupta et al., 2012).

The study described in this chapter explores and discusses intimate partner violence (IPV), marital conflict, domestic and family violence (DFV) through data collected from community leaders. It examines the perspectives and points of view of the community leaders about what further steps should be taken to prevent and to deal with IPV in post-genocide Rwandan society.

Methods of Research

Participants

The participants in the study who joined focus group discussions (FGDs) or provided individual interviews were local leaders and community-based workers who dealt with IPV, gender issues, and child protection and human rights affairs in their daily activities. The invitation to participate in the research was presented at the district level by the staff representative of the Ministry of Gender and Family Promotion who worked most closely with each prospective research participant; this approach helped by communicating official support for the study. Each focus group was composed of some of the following members at the district level: a representative of the Access to Justice Bureau; a representative of the National Women's Council; a community health worker; a staff member responsible for citizen registration; a land officer; a staff member in charge of good governance; people holding gender focal point positions; representatives of faith-based organizations and of the "guardian angels"[1]; a representative of *Haguruka* [Stand Up], a local non-governmental organization offering legal support to vulnerable children and women; and a representative of *Pro-Femmes/Twese hamwe* [Pro-Women Together], which is an umbrella organization working for the advancement of women, peace, and development in Rwanda.

Individual interviews with key informants were conducted with representatives of stakeholders of the GMO (Gender Monitoring Office) and other public and civil society organizations. Each of the following institutions was represented in the interviews: the Access to Justice Bureau,

---

[1] In 2007 the Imbuto Foundation, chaired by the First Lady of Rwanda, Jeannette Kagame, initiated a network called *Malayika Murinzi* [Guardian Angels] in order to create a protective environment for children who do not have appropriate care by promoting adoption and foster care.

the National Public Prosecution Authority, the National Police, the National Women's Council, the National Human Rights Commission, faith-based organizations, community-based organizations, the GMO, and the Ministry of Gender and Family Promotion. Both focus group discussions and individual interviews were conducted in the Nyamasheke District of Western Province, and in the Nyaruguru and Huye Districts of Southern Province.

A total of twenty-two people including twelve males and ten females participated in the three FGDs. Eleven people including eight males and three females participated in ten individual interviews. In one interview, two people working in the same office for prevention of IPV chose to participate together, as they wanted to complement each other in giving their views. Districts were represented by letters A (Nyamasheke), B (Nyaruguru), and C (Huye) in the data presentation and in the discussion.

As Table 8.1 shows, the gender distribution of the participants included more males than females (twelve males and eight females in the FGDs; eight males and thre females for the individual interviews). This reflects the actual gender distribution at the time of data collection among those occupying the roles in the areas of interest of the research: local leaders and community-based workers who dealt with IPV, gender issues, child protection, and human rights affairs in their daily activities, as well as representatives of stakeholders of the GMO and other public and civil society organizations.

Table 8.1 Number of participants in FGDs and in individual interviews

Place/district	Males in FGD	Females in FGD	Males in interviews	Females in interviews
District A	7	3	3	0
District B	2	4	2	1
District C	3	3	3	2
Total	12	10	8	3
Total number of participants in FGDs: 12 + 10 = 22			Total number of participants in individual interviews: 8 + 3 = 11	

The Research Approach

Interview and focus group discussion guides were developed in relation to the following research questions.

1. What is your understanding of intimate partner violence?
2. What are the different forms of intimate partner violence perpetrated in your district?
3. Are all cases of intimate partner violence reported?
4. What is the gender distribution of the victims? Who are the victims and perpetrators (men, women, or both)?
5. What strategies do you suggest should be put in place in order to combat intimate partner violence?

A moderator (the present author) and a note-taker (a research assistant) together conducted the three FGDs (one at the headquarters of each of the three districts) and the ten individual interviews with key informants. Ethical considerations of participation and confidentiality in research with human beings as participants were complied with. Participation was freely consented to and confidentiality was respected. Participants were not identifiable as research subjects in their workplaces because they participated in the study very much as part of their daily routine. From the outside a meeting with us looked like any other meeting, albeit somewhat longer so that we could cover the interview questions in our guide. To preserve confidentiality, participants' names were not mentioned in the collected data. FGDs and individual interviews were recorded with the permission of the participants. All the discussions were convivially conducted.

Analysis Techniques

The recoded data from the FGDs and individual interviews were transcribed and translated from Kinyarwanda into English. Thematic content analysis, a process for systematically examining text data using codes to facilitate retrieval of similar information across the data, was conducted (Miles & Huberman, 1994; Rubin & Rubin, 1995, 2005). First, the analysis considered the data from the FGDs separately from the data from the interviews. Throughout the analysis process, the location of the information given by the participants was recorded along with each of the identified themes and subthemes related to the research questions and objectives (Baribeau, 2009; Duchesne & Haegel, 2005; L'Ecuyer, 1989, 1990). Codes were compiled into subcategories, then compared, and combined into broader categories. Second, the analysis of the FGDs yielded themes and ideas corresponding to each question; these were grouped with similar themes and ideas for the same question from the individual interviews for use in the report presentation and discussion.

Results and Discussion

Understanding IPV

In both FGDs and interviews, participants spoke about their understanding of IPV. For them, IPV was an act of violence conducted by one spouse against the other, an act that inflicted harm and deprived the victimized spouse of their human rights.

> For me, intimate partner violence is when spouse, husband or wife, is deprived of his or her rights by the other. (FGD in C, female)

> I think it is any act done by someone to harm his or her partner. (FGD in A, male)

> I understand this as an act of depriving one's partner of his or her rights; it is harming one's spouse. (FGD in B, male)

> For me, it is violence committed against a partner, a man against his wife and vice versa. (Interview in A, male)

> For me, it is a violence committed in violating the rights of a person against his intimate partner. (Interview in C, male)

> It is a violation of the rights of the woman or of the man, but the definition must be consulted in accordance with the law. (Interview in C, female)

The participants' understanding of IPV fits with the WHO definition, which states that IPV "violates the fundamental rights of the victims" (García-Moreno et al., 2013; Krug et al., 2002).

Forms of IPV

Physical Violence

Physical harms—beating and in other ways harming the body—of one partner by the other was identified by participants as a type of IPV present in Rwanda.

> There are perpetrators who beat their victims, mainly the wives, and harm their body. Beating or harming the body is intimate partner violence. (FGD in B, male)

> There are times when the husband beats his wife and hurts her so that she has to go to the hospital. (FGD in B, female)

> To all the other types of violence cited discussed so far, I would add another type which is to harm the body, such as burning the body of one's spouse or other action to physically harm the body. (FGD in C, female)

Physical intimate partner violence is not particular to Rwanda; previous studies have included physical violence as a category of IPV in other countries as well (Ganley & Schechter, 1996; Krug et al., 2002).

Economic Violence

Participants identified several kinds of economic IPV, such as: no agreement between intimate partners on the uses of economic goods, lack of access to family income by one of the intimate partners, and the exclusive management or use of shared property by one of the intimate partners (usually the man).

> Spouses' disagreements on the uses of the economic goods they have in common often lead to constant harassment of one by the other. (FGD in A, male)

> The two spouses can be both civil servants and earning wages, but the husband puts himself in a position of being the head of everything, to the point where the woman, even to be able to buy salt or sanitary napkins, has to beg for it from her husband. The two partners are entitled to their wages, but the woman finds herself in a position of dependency. (FGD in B, female)

> Often women work very hard for the economic production, but the outcome of their efforts is not managed equitably by both men and women. The woman is not entitled to know the financial proceeds from the sale of their common goods. Even to have access to the property to be mortgaged can be impossible even though that property was acquired by both of them. (FGD in B, female)

> There are partners (mostly women) who do not have access to family income and property. Thus, the lack of access to family income and to property is intimate partner violence. (Interview in A, male)

> Apart from the cases that we receive here, from information we have seen on television, we realize that in the countryside, women are the victims, they have no wage labor and the conflicts and violence taking place there are mainly related to economic affairs. (Interview in C, female)

> The intimate partner violence is mainly based on economic aspects. Men are perpetrators against their wives and women are perpetrators against

their husbands. About 99.9% of the complaints we receive in our daily activities are economic, especially land-related. (Interview in B, male)

Previous studies agreed that issues related to economic exclusion, such as economic coercion of one partner by the other, are a type of IPV (Bragg, 2003; Ganley & Schechter, 1996; García-Moreno et al., 2013). Systematic gender inequality in Africa is often reinforced by cultural traditions that place men in the role of head of the household in charge of family finances and decisions (Bowman, 2003).

Killing of the Intimate Partner

Participants in this study were aware that some people are killed by their intimate partners. Such a death seems to be understood as a catastrophic human behavior toward the intimate partner, going beyond the other physical aspects of IPV because it makes an end to the victim's life.

Physical violence can end in the murder of one of the intimate partners, the man killing the woman or the woman killing the husband. (FGD in A, male)

Death due to killing is intimate partner violence; there are victims who are killed, murdered by their intimate partners; killers are mainly men. (FGD in C, male)

Murder of intimate partners is seen as a new phenomenon in Rwanda. According to a report released by the Rwanda National Police (IGIHE, 2017), forty-five women and nineteen men were killed by their spouses in 2016. In 2011, 121 women were murdered by their husbands, and ninety-one men were murdered by their wives (MIGEPROF, 2011a, 2011b). Even if these numbers appear to be not especially high given the Rwandan population of 12,374,397 (NISR, 2020), one might argue that even a single such case of murder is too many. The murder of one intimate partner by the other is a serious problem not just in Rwanda but around the world (Molinié, 2016; United Nations Office on Drugs and Crime, 2013).

The World Health Organization (2013) identifies IPV as an epidemic one that can be fatal. Thirty-eight percent of all murdered women were killed by their intimate partners (García-Moreno et al., 2013). There are as yet no studies showing clearly the reasons for intimate partner killings in Rwanda. Rubanzana et al. (2015) conducted a study of risk factors for homicide victimization in post-genocide Rwanda. They state that homicide victims tend to be relatively young and that the proportion of female victims is one of the highest in the world (Rubanzana et al., 2015). These authors argue that even in the context of residual effects from a mass genocide, homicide victimization risk factors are not unique to Rwanda. Thus, further research on the factors contributing to killings as one type of IPV in Rwanda would be of great interest.

Sexual Violence and Sexual Forcing

Participants described several forms of sexual violence, mainly involving men who forced their female partners into unwanted sexual relations. The participants regarded this as a form of rape, with consequences such as injury to the sexual body areas of the victim. Some spoke of men who felt that their payment of a dowry to the wives' families justified their making use of their wives' bodies as and when they saw fit, even when the women were not physically or psychologically ready.

> When there is a disagreement on sexual practices between spouses, or forcing, generally by men, in unwanted sexual relations, rape, and harm on the sexual body parts—that is intimate partner violence. (FGD in B, male)

> There are spouses who do not communicate before intercourse, which ends up creating conflict between the spouses. The husband can tell his wife that as he gave the dowry to have it, he can dispose of his wife's body as and when he…wants. (FGD in A, male)

> The husband may think that he is the chief or master of sexual relations with his wife; the one who has the say over it, and that the woman must show submission whenever the husband feels like it. Whether the woman

feels like it or not, her husband's wishes become an imperative to be followed and complied with. (FGD in B, female)

In my routine activities, I learn that there are some men who practice unusual and harmful sexual relations. This happens after those men have learned different unusual sexual practices from outside, such as in prison, and want to practice what has been acquired on their wives. Negatively surprised, the victim comes to me saying that she wants to leave her partner because he has changed. (FGD in B, female)

There are participants who spoke of men going beyond the traditions and laws that placed them at the "head of the household" to thinking that they were the master in all aspects of life, including sexual relations.

Men go beyond the traditional law that gave to them the right to be called the [head of the household] and use it in forcing sexually their wives while these wives are not in normal conditions, either they are tired or sick and then they are not in a situation to agree to sexual relations. (Interview in A, male)

On this point of heading the household, it is encouraging to note that a new household management scheme was recently put in place in Rwanda. It specifies that spouses jointly provide management including moral and material support to the household, and also provide for its maintenance (Republic of Rwanda, 2016). As the public become familiar with this law, it may contribute to a change in the mindset of men with regard to the power relation between them and their intimate partners.

Psychological and Spiritual Violence

Participants identified different types of psychological IPV, including harassment, degrading language, putting the victim in a position of suffering, lack of care towards a partner, forcing adherence to a set of spiritual practices, obliging a female partner to wait without sleep for the male's return until late at night, irresponsibility in supporting wives in domestic activities, polygamy, and harassing of wives because of the sex of the baby she gives birth to. On the other side, however, some participants felt that women who indulge in activities such as watching movies rather than taking care of their husbands should be considered when discussing IPV.

> Conjugal harassment may consist of degrading language or other action directed at the psychological suffering of the victim. There are victims of harassment who sleep outside the house, and the next day they go about their activities like everything is okay, nothing bad happened to them, they do not report officially, but only talk about it among them as ladies. (FGD in B, female)

> There is absence of care toward men by women spending lot of time in the night watching series films on television while the husband is waiting for her in the bedroom very late in the night. (FGD in C, male)

> There are husbands who harass wives because of giving birth to only one sex. (FGD in B, male)

> Can you imagine? I know an unfortunate case of intellectual spouses. Imagine that one is a lawyer who knows the laws, his wife is an economist. Do you know what they have for disagreement? This is because the woman bears only daughters! So, if an intellectual can say this how do you think that will be the situation for the people who are not intellectuals, living in the countryside?…I asked the following question to this man: "Do you know that it is the man who gives the sex of the child; do not you know that at least through the books?" He did not answer my question; he kept silent, now they are separated when they had three girls together! (FGD in C, male)

> We see intimate partner violence in religion, where the husband forces his wife to be in his faith orientation. For example, two people may marry but have different religions. After marriage, the husband may forcibly require his wife to join him in his own belief church. (FGD in B, male)

> There are men who, when they are outside the home during the night, oblige their wives to wait for them until they come. The wives are obliged by their husbands to wait for them and are not allowed to sleep before

the husband comes even if it is very late in the night. To me that is a type of intimate partner violence. (Interview in C, female)

There are irresponsible spouses, especially men, who do not take care of nor support their wives in domestic activities. (Interview in A, male)

Not helping women with the household chores is a form of intimate partner violence. (Interview in B, male)

Polygamy is a great problem that ends sometimes in the abandonment of one spouse—the previous one—for another. Such a situation happens especially when a spouse wants to be with another partner who seems to be richer than the previous partner. (Interview in A, male)

Psychological and spiritual violence are unhealthy, and amount to a public health problem. The World Health Organization (Krug et al., 2002) includes psychological harm as a category of intimate partner violence.

Extent of Reporting of Cases of IPV

Gender Aspect of the Victim in Reporting IPV

Women are said to report incidents of IPV much more often than men. As one participant stated:

In terms of gender reporting, women are the main victims who report about intimate partner violence and the CNF [National Women's Council] helps in this. Men do not, maybe because of their culture they do not want to let it be known that they are victims of their partners. They do not want to be seen as victims of females. (FGD in A, female)

Types of IPV Reported

IPV is not always reported as soon as it happens. Often, the victim herself is not able to report her own case; rather, the help of someone who can advocate for the victim is required. The psychological suffering of the victim is not disclosed unless it has resulted in physical consequences. Unlike psychological violence, economic violence is generally reported by the victims, and again these are mainly women.

> Especially when it is a case of sexual intimate partner violence, female victims are the ones who report their cases. But note also that, even so, women do it only when the situation has already become intolerable. Intimate partner violence cases are not automatically reported; they are not reported as soon as they happen. (FGD in A, male)

> When it comes to types of intimate partner violence, sexual violence is not systematically reported. When it is sexual intimate partner violence, victims start by telling it to a confidante. Then this confidante may advise the victim to report to the MAJ[2] or to police. The victim cannot take the initiative of reporting his or her own case: this needs the help of the CNF or of anyone who can help in doing advocacy for the victim about the violence faced. (FGD in A, male)

> Intimate partner harassment, which may consist of degrading language or other action aimed at the psychological suffering of the victim, is not disclosed, it is not put out, and it is not reported. This type of intimate partner violence becomes known only in the case of extreme physical consequences of injury or death of the victim...there are those who are victims of harassment who do not tell the authorities, there are some who are forced to sleep outside the house; the next day they go to their activities as if nothing had happened. (FGD in B, female)

> The harassment between intimate partners that may be of the man against his wife or wife against her husband is not said, it is not reported. This is different from when the cases are related to economic violence. Women who are the main victims of economic violence now know that they can be assisted if, for example, the husband has unilaterally sold an economic good, the victim goes to the authority and denounces the husband's

---

[2]MAJ means (in French) *Maison d'Accès à la Justice* [House of Access to Justice]; it is a service whereby people are freely assisted with legal services in Rwanda.

action and asks for advice on the procedure to follow for this violence to be resolved. (FGD in B, male)

I feel it is hard. I, who live in the countryside, I see that the situation is complicated for the woman who lives there in the countryside. The woman who lives in the countryside has a baby on her back, sometimes she is even pregnant, and she went to the field with her husband if she is lucky enough to be accompanied by him for the work. Being back at a house, the husband asks the woman for food while they have both just arrived at home, having been working together in the field for agricultural activities...Even if the husband beats her, she must be silent; she must not denounce her husband, for fear of not being able to escape. She thinks that if her husband sends her away, she will not have a place to go, especially since even her own parents, especially her mother informs her that this is how marital life works, that the difficult situation must be kept as it happens. So she lives in that situation...the woman who lives in the countryside is a victim of especially economic violence. She works a lot for conjugal and family production, but her share of the product of her work is limited. (FGD in B, female)

Not all victims report themselves. Many of the victims keep silent about intimate partner violence because the culture tells them that it is normal to live in such a situation of being violated by their husbands. Because of the influence of culture, many cases are not said; many keep silent because they say: "*niko zubakwa* [that's how homes work]"! (FGD in C, male)

Cases of intimate partner violence we are aware of in our hospital services are those which ended in physical violence, or in transmissible diseases; they are generally sent to us by the police. (Interview in A, male)

Other Factors Inhibiting the Reporting of IPV

Other factors that may keep a victim from reporting IPV are the psychosocial environment, intimidation of the victim, and the insufficient quality of the client care received from the people who handle reports of IPV, especially the lack of normal follow-up on the reported cases.

> Reporting intimate partner violence is a very delicate situation. The administration is making efforts against intimate partner violence, but the result is not tangible. The victims are intimidated by the perpetrators who tell them that if they denounce them, they will kill them. Thus, the victims look at the consequences that they incur when denouncing the violence of which they are victims and choose to not report. (FGD in C, male)

> The way victims are helped may discourage other victims from telling about their case. There are people who receive the victims in bad ways which are not in accordance with the situation of the intimate partner violence. (FGD in C, female)

> Reporting intimate partner violence also depends on how those who state their cases are accompanied and helped. I think there are problems here. I will give you an example. I once accompanied a woman who had been dangerously beaten by her intimate partner. When the victim arrived at the police station, a woman who was also at the police station at that time and who knew the victim said, "But why is this woman rushing to report the violence she is suffering from when she is not married legally with the man?" The police officer, who heard the reaction of that woman, took that opportunity to ask the victim, "Madam, are you not married legally?" and the victim replied that she was not. So the policeman said, "Well, be beaten to death, you whore!"...Imagine the situation that had just been created, and that mother who had just been called a whore rather than being assisted on the acts of violence...Fortunately the commander arrived at that moment and, observing the victim, he sympathized, and the situation became more or less relaxed...The way in which the victims are helped is problematic: Rwandans in general think that women can be beaten by their partners. (FGD in C, female)

> There are also times when repeated acts of violence take place and the local authority who receives repeated complaints from the same victim comes to have had enough, and can say to the victim, "But we help you and you do not stop your violence." This seems as if the situation

of violence does not finally have definitive solutions and it is probably discouraging for the victim. (FGD in C, male)

We sometimes lack a model in the handling of intimate partner violence cases. Sometimes, you report the case of violence at the administrative sector level, but sometimes the person you're addressing yourself to does the same thing: he lives in the intimate partner violence situation. What help can that person bring? I do have a proposal: The counselors should be numerous because everyone is sick...the reactions we see today shown on children, on men, on women...They missed psychosociological assistance, they missed having someone to listen to them, and their situations degenerated. Permanent counseling is needed. (FGD in C, female)

Adequate support and follow-up of reported cases and support to victims is an issue. That is what I observe and it grieves me much. Follow-up of cases: reported cases have no appropriate follow-up system. I do not know if this is because there are no consequences against the authority that does not take appropriate action on the case that is reported. I do not know whether this is due to the fact that he is not a model, or that he does not care about this case, or the fact that it may be due to the lack of knowledge about intimate partner violence. There are reported cases that are not treated, but are classified by the one who should follow it up...There is no follow-up system that I know of. I am now in my third term as women's representative...but I do not know any follow-up system. For example, one [official] can receive a case: he promises that this problem will be followed up and that stops there, nothing else is done after there. At one point after, we hear that a victim has just been killed, or a girl has just thrown her baby in the toilet; there are many reactions when cases of intimate partner violence are not followed up. The woman we visited at the hospital had been burned by her husband by pouring a pot of potatoes on her face, she was burned on her face, on her breasts, but I tell you the truth, it has not had any continuation. (FGD in C, female)

I learned that he asked for forgiveness and that he received it. (FGD in C, female)

I too learned that he was forgiven by the police and that is all. This kind of person—a professional who interceded for forgiveness when he was the one who would have punished the crime—should be answering this, he should be accountable to this. (FGD in C, female)

Several factors influence whether an IPV incident will be reported. The gender of the victim plays a role. Most of the victims who report IPV are female. Men tend not to report, perhaps due to the influence of their culture. Men may deny being victims to avoid being known as the victims of females. This is consistent with the findings of Umubyeyi et al. (2014), who, with regard to men's lower reporting rate, stated that men's denial of incidents could be explained by the gender role pattern.

Sexual and economic violence are the types of IPV most likely to be reported. Sexual abuse by a partner is more often reported by female than by male victims, but the reporting is not automatic, nor does it usually take place immediately. Instead, the female victims tend to keep silent until the situation has become more and more catastrophic and reaches a breaking point. They take rarely the initiative on their own to report, but need support from other people, especially from organizations dedicated to women's development such as CNF (*Conseil National des Femmes* [National Council of Women]) and from any person in a position to advocate for the victim. Indeed, consistent with the present findings, it has been reported that only 42% of women who have ever experienced physical or sexual violence sought help from either formal or informal sources; the majority of women preferred informal sources of help, such as family, in-laws, friends, or neighbors (Umubyeyi et al., 2016). However, while the present study found that in order for female victims of IPV to report they need the assistance and support of others, Thomson et al. (2015), in a study on correlates of IPV against women during a time of rapid social transition in Rwanda, analyzed the 2005 and 2010 Rwanda Demographic and Health Surveys and found that Rwanda has one of the highest self-reported rates of IPV against women worldwide, and that multiple forms of current or past violence are reported by the same women. This suggests a need for further studies on the conditions leading to cases of IPV being reported.

The victims of economic violence are usually female, and there is less reluctance to report this type of IPV. Intimate partner harassment, on the other hand, is not generally reported to authorities. This type of IPV is usually recognized only when it leads to extreme physical consequences of injury or death of the victim. Cultural influences play an important part in the underreporting of cases, especially in the countryside, where women are less educated. Female victims are exhorted to live with the IPV they suffer from because, as the saying goes, "*niko zubakwa* [that is how homes work]." For male victims, it is not culturally easy to accept and reveal that the male is the victim of a female intimate partner.

Other factors also play a role in discouraging the reporting of IPV. These relate to the psychosocial environment and intimidation of the victims by the perpetrators. If the perpetrators tell the victims that if they denounce them, they will be killed, the victims will probably choose not to report. This is consistent with the statement that women feared revealing abuse to anyone, either within or outside the family, as this would bring shame to the family and worsen their overall life situation (Umubyeyi et al., 2016). Umubyeyi and colleagues recommended that a study be carried out on gaps in legislation aimed at supporting abused women; they also suggested the need for a study on gaps in the involvement of health care professionals in supporting abused women (2016).

Untrained or insufficiently trained staff, or staff whose moral values negatively impact their relationships with the victims, will lead to unsatisfactory client care and will handicap the reporting of IPV cases. It is of great importance that professionals who deal with IPV cases should receive the right training to develop the needed skills. Previous authors have made similar recommendations. For example, in the medical aspect of IPV, Umubyeyi et al. (2016) recommended that health care professionals should be better prepared through further education, and guidelines on how to handle such cases.

With regard to reported cases of IPV, Thomson et al. (2015) conducted an analysis of the 2005 and 2010 demographic and health surveys. They concluded that there had been a doubling in self-reported violence between 2005 and 2010, and that it coincided with major political and social gains in Rwanda. However, they also recommended that additional research be conducted to tease out to what extent increased self-reports of IPV are due to increased IPV incidence rather than greater empowerment by women to report violence. They also stated that research is needed to evaluate the effectiveness of IPV interventions such as police station gender desks and district hospital Isange [Feel Welcome] One Stop Centers[3] in reducing the incidence of IPV (Thomson et al., 2015).

Participants suggested that good follow-up of reported cases is necessary in order to avoid extreme consequences, such as death. There is a need to expand the number of locations where justice services can be accessed, so that in each two or three administrative sectors there are justice services to support victims in the local area. There is a need for psychologists at police offices and for a multidisciplinary team to deal with IPV. As Bragg (2003) suggested, this could be beneficial in such areas as crisis counseling and interventions, support groups, medical and mental health referrals, legal advocacy, vocational counseling, and children's services.

The Status and Gender Distribution of Victims and Perpetrators of IPV

Participants felt that children were incontestably victims of IPV. When asked to rank the main victims of IPV by importance, they put children first, women second, and men third. This is apparent from the FGD and interview data, but also from the energy that was put into talking about the issue of victims of IPV. Participants unanimously reported that the victims of IPV include both female and male partners, and that the children of violent intimate partners are collateral victims. When discussing "who are the victims" of IPV, both nonverbal behaviors and the tone of the conversation clearly showed the insistence of the participants that

---

[3] Isange one stop center (IOSC) use holistic model and multidisciplinary approach in terms of the provision of medical, legal, forensic/investigation, psychosocial and safety needs to help victims of violence and child abuse, the majority of whom are women and girls. https://rwanda. un.org/en/15872-rwandas-holistic-approach-tackling-different-faces-gender-based-violence-gbv.

children and women are the main victims of IPV, with men in third place.

> Children are the main victims of intimate partner violence. In terms of gender of the victims of intimate partner violence, both men and women are victims. (FGD in A, male)

> When I look at it, I realize that children are the first victims. A child who lives in a marital home where there is IVP, he gets hurt psychologically, fails to be properly educated by his parents. Then he will not be able to properly follow his lessons at school. He grows up in an environment of conflict...When he sees that his parents are still fighting, he may think that when the day comes when he will have his own marital home, the situation will be the same, which puts him in a situation of [psychological discomfort]. (FGD in C, female)

> To me, victims of intimate partner violence are women and children. Even if the female was the perpetrator of the intimate partner violence, her nature as a female means that she also became the victim of the situation she created herself. (FGD in A, female)

> To me, whether the intimate partner violence is perpetrated by men or by women, the victims are children and women; if I try to make a kind of proportion, I can say that 90 percent of victims are women and children, and only 1 or 2 percent of victims of intimate partner violence are male. (FGD in B, male)

> The victims of intimate partner violence are first children, women second, and men third. But this depends on the perpetrator of the intimate partner violence. (FGD in A, male)

> Here in our district, if I compare it with other districts I've worked in, I realize that it all depends on the district...I have tangible cases where both sides are undergoing intimate partner violence. Intimate partner violence is not committed against women only; men also come and tell us that they are the victims of intimate partner violence by their wives. Women give a mistaken interpretation of gender equality: she now knows that she is the equal of man. As the man approaches her, she calls the police

saying her husband has just beaten her and the rumors are circulating as well...Today, there are men who have made the decision to leave the domestic home leaving their wives behind them...The reference I can give you is that in about four requests for divorce, one can be by a man. (FGD in B, female)

Women are the main victims. Yes, there are some cases of men who are victims, but the majority of victims of intimate partner violence are women, and most of the perpetrators are men. (Interview in A, male)

Most of the time, the victims of intimate partner violence are women. The reason for this is that, generally speaking, in the Rwandan mentality, the husband is the head of all...But with regard to the new law of the family on the two spouses as chiefs...he may want to use conjugal economic assets as he wishes, unbeknownst to the woman. So if the woman presents resistance to her husband, she ends up being violated by him. It is in this way that the violence begins. (Interview in B, male)

But there are also women who want to seize and use only matrimonial goods, under the pretext that the law protects them. (Interview in A, male)

Women and girls are the main victims of IPV, and children are the main victims of the consequences of intimate partner violence. We regularly face these types of violence. Even when we do interventions with people who are facing intimate partner violence, we want to help mainly their children. (Interview in C, female)

Children and women are said to be the main victims of IPV. Men are said to be the usual perpetrators even if they also are sometimes victims. This finding about the gender of the victims and perpetrators of IPV is consistent with Umubyeyi and colleagues' (2014) study conducted in rural and urban areas of Rwanda's Southern Province. The authors found that both men and women were exposed to IPV, although men to a considerably lesser extent than women. IPV exposure, in the form of repeated acts of physical, sexual, and psychological violence, was commonly faced by women, while men reported only single incidents of violence.

In sub-Saharan Africa, women are more exposed to IPV than men (Were et al., 2011). Men report less exposure to physical and sexual violence while psychological violence exposure is more evenly distributed, irrespective of the time span under investigation—for example, the past year, or a lifetime (see, e.g., Nybergh et al., 2012). Some researchers have suggested that female victims are also often perpetrators of violence and that the victim and perpetrator roles can be played by both men and women (see, e.g., Bélanger et al., 2013). While it is true that IPV is perpetrated by both women and men, the majority of cases worldwide are perpetrated by males against their female partners (García-Moreno et al., 2013).

IPV is not only a matter of spouses or of two people in intimate relationship; it also has a harsh impact with negative physical and psychological outcomes on children (Doyle & McWilliams, 2018). In this regard, intimate partner violence may be a domestic and family violence (DFV), because its consequences affect all the family/household members. Even if domestic and family violence (DFV) is a serious issue globally, experienced by individuals from all backgrounds and societies (Doyle & McWilliams, 2018), women and children in post-conflict communities are at greatest risk (Bradley, 2018). Intimate partner violence (IPV) or destructive marital conflict or domestic and family violence (DFV) can be experienced by both women and men, but studies show that the majority of violence and abuse in relationships is from men to women (Breiding et al., 2014; Department of Justice, 2013).

Proposed Strategies Against IPV: Effective Preventive Measures

Participants suggested a number of measures as effective preventive and responsive actions for IPV. These include fighting against poverty, educating and sensitizing family members about their responsibilities and community leaders about laws and human rights, involving the churches in the fight against IPV by promoting mutual respect, training and educating people about gender equality and IPV, increasing the access to social services, reducing the distance to access help in cases of IPV, and improving telephone and other communications facilities. They also proposed putting in place a law discouraging and protecting free unions, the creation of a specific institution in charge of IPV, premarital education, adequate follow-up of reported cases and supporting of victims, and the punitive response.

Fighting Against Poverty

> A woman who does not make economic inputs to the home, even if she is in charge of rural field work and other domestic activities, she is not given value in the home. (FGD in C, female)

> Women do not yet have the same economic resources as men…They have begun to make economic contributions to their homes, but they have not yet reached the same level as men. (FGD in C, female)

> We see many people living in poverty. So when the wife asks her husband for something while the husband does not have the financial means to satisfy his wife's request, both spouses begin to denigrate each other. I think fighting poverty would be a solution to the intimate partner violence related to the impossibility of meeting the economic needs. (Interview in C, male)

In their study, Umubyeyi et al. (2014) also suggested that income-generating activities and access to financial credit would contribute to women's empowerment.

Educating and Sensitizing Family Members About Their Responsibilities and Community Leaders About Laws and Human Rights

Educating men and women so that everyone knows about their conjugal duties...the man has the responsibility to produce for and protect the home...The solution is to try to educate...Our contribution as a church is to educate. At least my son understands who the woman is, and who the man is. This is to avoid that, as we have seen that children are the first victims of intimate partner violence, that if they see their father beating their mothers, these children do not think that this is how it should be. (FGD in C, male)

It is important that the laws are explained to the people who are the beneficiaries. The laws are potentially good, they come to regulate marital and family problems, but people do not have the same interpretations regarding the laws. Men and women, and even children, must have the same understanding and interpretations of the law governing the family. The laws are not explained in ordinary language, laws are not sufficiently disseminated...You see that there are even intellectuals who act badly, more than those who are not educated...When the laws are not explained to the population, this creates difficulties...It is said that a law has gone out in the *Gazette*...but how many read the *Gazette*? Laws are good, but lack of awareness about them by beneficiaries is a problem. (FGD in C, female)

I agree with the same point, it is urgent to educate and explain the laws on the family...To speak on radio and television is not enough...Even among those who listen to the radio or watch television...many are interested in other shows like football. (FGD in C, male)

At the village level, to educate people on the contents of various laws about the human protection. (FGD in A, male)

There is a need for sensitization of local government...and the population on human rights. (FGD in B, male)

It is important to educate people about their rights. Someone may be confronted with intimate partner violence and believe that their torturer has the right to do so. It is important to know their rights and to know how to seek help in the case of intimate partner violence in order to claim rights when they are baffled. (Interview in B, male)

We must continue to raise awareness so that people know the rights of others. This is because, for example, there are men who believe that all rights belong to them, forgetting that women have rights also. (Interview in C, male)

It is necessary to educate the population on the right way to live. They should also be made aware of the types of intimate partner violence. A woman can publicly denigrate her husband and the husband does not know that this is a form of intimate partner violence. This affects the harmony of their life. (Interview in A, male)

Since they have not learned this at school, it is necessary that local authorities should be educated about intimate partner violence. In turn, these local authorities have to educate, to sensitize the population about intimate partner violence. (Interview in A, male)

Educational awareness on gender equality and human rights issues would contribute to women's empowerment. (Umubyeyi et al., 2014)

Involving the Churches in the Fight Against IPV by Promoting Mutual Respect

Churches should help people to change and family members to be patient with each other. (FGD in C, male)

In addition to the existing administrative institutions and the specific body dealing specifically with intimate partner violence, churches would help to educate the faithful on the fact that no one among intimate partners is an angel. (Interview in C, female)

Training and Educating People About Gender Equality and IPV

The gender concept needs to be well understood: men think that gender [equality] is only to the advantage of women and causes women not to respect those men. Men say that gender gives power to women. (FGD in B, male)

Increasing Access to Social Services, Reducing the Distance to Access Help in Cases of IPV, and Upgrading Telephone and Other Communications Facilities

To increase MAJ so that each two or three administrative sectors should have a MAJ service near the population. (FGD in A, male)

People travel long distances to reach police stations and MAJ services. For example, you see we are now at 10 a.m., but it is possible that someone who is coming here may be still on his way to here. It would be good to make available at least more than one bureau of MAJ, at least one MAJ bureau for two administrative sectors. However, it is necessary to sensitize the population about the opportunity they have…to use the calling way [a free telephone call] to police stations in order to report cases and get assistance. (Interview in A, male)

Proposing a Law Both Discouraging and Protecting Free Unions

There should be a law discouraging and protecting free relational unions. For people who live without being legally married, there is a form of instability that takes place in them and which influences their lives. This instability makes neither partner feel responsible for their household. Why cannot we decide by law that if a couple who are not legally married has spent a certain amount of time together, the household will be legally recognized as a home? We need to protect these families…This is a problem we often hear about...here. Every year we officially legalize illegal relationships, there is nothing preventing these types of disorderly relationships. Thus, if a man has decided to live with a girl, thinking that this is only a way for him to acquire the satisfaction of his sexual enjoyments, he has to feel engaged in responsibilities, that it will not be easy to get rid of her should he wish it. And for the girl, she will have to understand that if she engages in this type of relationship, it involves responsibilities and that if she has spent a certain time with that man, he will be her legal husband. (FGD in C, female)

I was in an administrative sector of our district. I had discussions with people in charge of the civil registry, community police, and so on. I asked them the following question: A young man and a girl decide to live together as husband and wife, how will you behave in this situation as a responsible action?...I addressed this question to about four people randomly chosen in the assembly and their answers were the same: we will try to hunt this strange girl...so understand that that girl becomes a victim of violence...I added another question: and if she ever became pregnant in the time she was with that man, what will become of the child she carries...All answered that he will be a street child... and you see, those are leaders...there were pastors, executive secretaries of the administrative cells, development officers at the level of the administrative unit...and we have conducted such discussions in all the administrative sectors...by bringing together all these categories of people...It is a problem, they said...but who can be sure that this pregnancy is not due to someone other than this young man? (FGD in C, female)

Proposing a Specific Institution to Address IPV

It would be helpful to set up a specific institution in charge of intimate partner violence so that it may be managed well, because it seems that in some existing institutions, intimate partner violence is given less importance...and this may be because there are more important problems for those institutions to handle. (Interview in C, female)

What I can propose is that there will be a specific body in charge of awareness and prevention of intimate partner violence. There should also be a specific law to punish intimate partner violence, for the population to become seriously aware of the problem of intimate partner violence. There should be a specific focus on intimate partner violence as there is, for example, a specific body for cases about trade. (Interview in B, male)

Undoubtedly, one can say that the problems [of intimate partner violence] do not resolve ...It is not easy to know exactly where the blocking is...many of them remain in suspense. At least, you never see someone saying that his intimate partner violence problems have found solutions at 100 percent...We think it would require a specific body dedicated to intimate partner violence and marital problems. I think that if intimate partner violence has not been solved as it is wished and wanted, maybe it is because the normal channels [of justice], which have to cope with varied problems of varied weights, can be overwhelmed if there are [many domestic violence cases] in addition to robbery and other serious crimes. When this happens, those other serious crimes receive much more attention; household crimes receive little importance if [the authorities] are involved in these other cases of crimes of particular gravity. This is the reason why we say that it could be fruitful if there was a specific body for solving conjugal problems. Existing institutions deal with many other crucial, important issues. When intimate partner violence cases arrive at police stations, in existing courts, and there are serious cases other than intimate partner violence, they [IPV cases] receive little attention beyond what is considered important in their [the courts] particular context. Just as there was a particular body that came to solve specific cases, the *Gacaca* [community justice court] came to solve specific problems of genocide and it was effective according to what was expected from them. A task force to deal with these domestic problems at the sector or district level, this would depend on the institutionalization, discussions focused on these problems; I think this may have good results, better than we see today. (Interview in C, female)

Premarital Education

What I can add on the topics of community education is, that there should be specific themes for those who are getting ready to get married...so that they understand the concept [of] gender...so that everybody marries knowing what awaits him in married life and what he will have to do in order to avoid annoying the other, his spouse. (FGD in C, female)

Premarital education should be conducted early and several times. There is a need for family counselors and for setting up a good methodology to improve education on family dynamics (living together). (Interview in C, male)

Adequate Follow-up of Reported Cases and Support of Victims

It would be helpful to follow up reported cases to avoid extreme consequences, such as death. (Interview in B, male)

There is a need for a psychologist at police stations, and there is a need for a multidisciplinary team that can make what is called a One Stop Center. (Interview in C, female)

Punitive Response

It would be important to consider intimate partner violence as a criminal act to be punished before the population in a public place. (FGD in B, male)

What I can add is that all intimate partner violence should be considered as criminal cases. We support the forgiveness that can be given by a victim of intimate partner violence, but there are no lessons that this can give to others...See for example that man overturning a boiling pot of sweet potatoes on his wife and sometime later, he said to his wife, "Pardon me, my wife, you know that we have children together"...and the victim forgives...In these conditions, another man will do the same thing because he will tell himself that women are like that, they are violated and they forgive. The perpetrator must be punished and the victim must be protected. (FGD in C, male)

I, too, would like to argue that intimate partner violence should be considered as criminal. The prosecution must recognize the value of forgiveness, but he should also recognize that forgiveness is not enough in cases of intimate partner violence, and that punishment is necessary. Intimate partner violence must be seen as criminal and punished as such. (FGD in C, male)

Discussion of the Proposed Strategies

One available preventive measure is that of addressing the problem of poverty. Although Rwanda has embarked on a policy of empowering women, they have not yet reached the same status as men. Thus some are still dependent on men financially. When women are obliged to beg money from their male partners, this may lead to underestimating the value of women as human beings. The value of women is sometimes estimated in terms of the income they can bring into the household.

Each intimate partner needs to be educated about his or her responsibilities in the relationship. It is important that children have good role models so that they will behave properly when they have their own households. The role of family education in preventing IPV is crucial.

The laws, especially the laws regulating the family, need to be explained to those who will benefit from them. Although a law may have the potential to do good, unless people at all levels of instruction and all degrees of social status know and understand the law, that potential will not be realized. Local leaders in particular and the population in general, need to become knowledgeable about IPV, human rights, and what steps to take when human rights are violated by IPV.

The concept of gender needs to be well explained, because there are men and women who misunderstand it. The misunderstanding of the gender concept can lead to inappropriate behaviors in a relationship between intimate partners. Rwandan psychosocial medical professionals have emphasized the importance of making the concept of gender well understood in order to prevent conflict and violence linked to misunderstanding of gender by men and by women (Mukashema & Sapsford, 2013). The need for education and sensitization as a measure to prevent family conflict leading to violence was also noted (Mukashema & Sapsford, 2013).

Religious institutions can help to prevent IPV by promoting attitudinal change and mutual patience among family members. Advocacy efforts such as public awareness campaigns, collaborating with community services providers, and efforts to secure safety for victims and their children (Bragg, 2003) can help raise awareness about IPV. To succeed, strategies to reduce partner violence need the combined commitment of all actors, such as government and civil society (Abramsky et al., 2011).

The helping services in cases of IPV, such as MAJ and police stations, should be as nearby and accessible to the population as possible. Rwanda has set up a communications strategy that allows IPV victims to report offenders with a free telephone call. Putting in place a law discouraging and protecting free relational unions, by giving them legal recognition after a period of cohabitation, would be good for the prevention of IPV against women and would especially benefit the children of those unions. Formal marriage needs to be emphasized as a protective factor against IPV (Abramsky et al., 2011).

The participants suggested that a specific institution in charge of IPV should be created. They felt that IPV is not given enough importance, perhaps because institutions that are handling IPV also handle other serious issues to which they give more weight. An institution focusing only on issues of IPV and domestic violence could reduce this problem. These important suggestions come at a time when there is an effort to address IPV already underway in Rwanda, with a number of laws formulated to this end. For example, in 2008, a law regarding the prevention and punishment of gender-based violence was put in place. In 2009, a One Stop Center project offering free, integrated medical, psychosocial, and legal services to victims of IPV and child abuse was created. Almost all police stations now staff a gender desk with trained, usually female, personnel in order to help victims of IPV and other forms of domestic violence. The need for such measures indicates that IPV in Rwanda is an alarming issue. Indeed, it impacts negatively on the family, the smallest social unit and the foundation of a normal and harmonious nation.

Participants emphasized the importance of sufficient time for premarital education for people wishing to get married. Premarital education was also suggested in a previous study as a method of preventing marital conflict in Rwanda (Mukashema & Sapsford, 2013). For the purpose of premarital education, there is a need for family counselors who would set up a methodology for education about family dynamics (living together) in Rwanda. This premarital and family education should protect the children from IPV. Abramsky et al. (2011) suggested that early experiences of abuse for children are a strong risk factor for IPV in adulthood. Protecting and supporting victims and their children is a necessary responsive action to IPV (Schechter, 2000).

All reported cases of IPV should be followed up to avoid extreme consequences, including death. A multidisciplinary team, consisting of staff well trained in handling IPV, should be in charge of the cases to ensure good and comprehensive client care and adequate support to victims. While the Rwandan health and legal sectors have multiple initiatives to support victims, additional campaigns may be needed to shift public perception and reduce perpetration of IPV (Thomson et al., 2015).

Even in recognizing the value of forgiveness in relationships, punishing IPV is needed as an example to other potential perpetrators. Participants believed that public punishment would discourage domestic violence. Suggested responsive actions to IPV from previous studies included improving the legal and criminal justice response (e.g., Schechter, 2000), accountability for perpetrators of IPV through societal and criminal sanctions, and systematic changes to combat IPV and to promote victims' rights (Bragg, 2003). Women who survive IPV feel more empowered to report by the protection provided by the laws, and, as a result, an increase in the number of arrests for non-lethal spousal violence has occurred (United Nations Office on Drugs and Crime, 2013).

IPV was understood by the participants in this study as an act characterized by the deprivation of spouses' rights and involving violence, physical or otherwise, by one spouse against the other. One noted, however, that the definition given by law must also be kept in mind. Physical IPV may consist of beating and harming the body of the victim, which can end in the death of the victim. The identified features of economic IPV are non-agreement between intimate partners on the uses of their economic goods; lack of access to family income by the victim, who is generally female; and the selfishness of the perpetrator in the management and the use of their common property. Sexual IPV consists mainly of unwanted sexual relations perpetrated by men. Some men think that the payment of a dowry to the wife's family confers on them the right to control their female intimate partners and even abuse them. Some also cling to the traditional male role as head of the family, with the right to dictate practices in the area of sexual relations. Psychological IPV includes harassment, degrading language, failing to take care of one's partner, imposing spiritual adherence, and the persecution of wives according to the sex of their babies, as well as irresponsibility in supporting the victims (generally the wives) in domestic activities.

Participants noted that the victims who report IPV are most often women. However, sexual violence frequently goes unreported. Victims may initially keep silent, and then make a report when the situation has become unbearable. Female victims of sexual violence generally need support from other people before they report. Economic violence is the form of IPV most readily reported by its victims, who are generally female. Harassment, on the other hand, is not generally reported to authorities, even though it may lead to a degenerating situation with extreme physical consequences including injury to or the death of the victim. To some extent, failure to report cases of IPV is influenced by culture, especially in the countryside, where women are less educated. They may be told by elders, especially their family members, that being violated for a wife is not unusual, and that it is simply how homes work (*niko zubakwa*).

Men generally do not report IPV. This is probably linked to traditional cultural influences that lead men to deny being the victim of a female intimate partner. The Rwandan government is making efforts against IPV, especially in raising awareness among victims of the benefit of reporting IPV, but the results are not yet tangible. Some factors that explain the underreporting of IPV include intimidation, the psychosocial environment, and the nature of client care. If the perpetrators tell the victims that if they denounce them, they will be killed, the victims will probably choose not to report the violence. Some issues relating to the quality of the client care obtained by victims from the people dealing with IPV, as well as the way reported cases are followed up, are said to be factors that discourage IPV reporting.

Participants proposed a number of measures aimed at preventing IPV, destructive marital conflict, and domestic and family violence: fighting against poverty, educating and sensitizing family members about their responsibilities and community leaders about laws and human rights, involving the churches in the fight against IPV by fostering mutual respect between family members, training and educating people about gender equality and IPV, increasing the access of people to the helping services and reducing the amount of travel required, implementing a law both discouraging and protecting free unions, creating a specific institution dedicated to IPV issues, engaging in premarital education, ensuring adequate follow-up of reported cases, and better support for victims. The criminal penalties for IPV should be strengthened and fully enforced in order to set an example that will inhibit new potential perpetrators.

Conclusion

This chapter emphasizes two important aspects about intimate partner violence (IPV). First, the main and collateral victims of IPV are the children, as the participants have stated. This means that IPV is not only an issue regarding partners in intimate relationship, but also it is rather an issue to the families at large, because it includes the children as victims. Post-conflict communities lack laws criminalizing acts of DFV (Bradley, 2018). This author suggests the development of legislation both criminalizing DFV and facilitating the legal protection of victims (Bradley, 2018). Studies have revealed that experiences and patterns of IPV are shaped by the social, political, cultural and economic factors that exist in a given society (Doyle & McWilliams, 2018).

Second, post-conflict societies consistently experience high rates of domestic and family violence (DFV) against women and children (Bradley, 2018). The current research as well as the previous one conducted in this domain in Rwanda show that like in other post-conflict societies, the problems of intimate partner violence (IPV), destructive marital conflict, domestic and family violence (DFV) are still there and is said to have increased in post-genocide Rwandans society (MIGEPROF, 2011a, 2011b; Mukashema & Sapsford, 2013; Ndushabandi et al., 2016; NISR, 2012; Rutayisire & Richters, 2014; Sarabwe et al., 2018; Umubyeyi et al., 2014).

The content of this chapter is consistent with the perspective that intimate partner violence, destructive marital conflict, together with domestic and family violence increase in post-conflict society in general and in post-genocide Rwandan society in a particular way. Thus, Rwanda is a new case illustrating the phenomenon of intimate partner violence (IPV) and domestic and family violence (DFV) in relation with conflict societies. However, further comparative research on pre- and post-genocide intimate partner violence (IPV), destructive marital conflict, and domestic and family violence (DFV) in Rwandan society would be of an important interest. Comparative research on pre- and post-genocide intimate partner violence (IPV), destructive marital conflict, domestic and family violence (DFV) in Rwandan society are suggested to be designed and implemented.

Acknowledgements This research was conducted through the facilitation of the Rwandan Gender Monitoring Office's research initiative. An earlier version of this chapter was published as: "A report about intimate partner violence in southern and western Rwanda" in the *International Journal of Child, Youth and Family Studies* (2017) 9(3), 68–99. https://doi.org/10.18357/ijcyfs932018 18277. A new analysis including the data's aspects of post-conflict societies as well as the marital conflict, domestic, and family aspects of IPV was conducted.

Declaration of Interest Statement
There is no conflict of interest.

References

Abramsky, T., Watts, C. H., Garcia-Moreno, C., Devries, K., Kiss, L., Ellsberg, M., Jansen, H. A. F. M., & Heise, L. (2011). What factors are associated with recent intimate partner violence? Findings from the WHO multi-county study on women's health and intimate partner violence. *BMC Public Health, 11*, 109. https://doi.org/10.1186/1471-2458-11-109.

American Psychiatric Association. (2013). *The diagnostic and statistical manual of mental disorders. 5th Edition. DSM-5.* Washington, DC.

Baribeau, C. (2009). Analyse des entretiens de groupe [Analysis of group interviews]. *Recherches Qualitatives, 28*(1), 133–148.

Bélanger, C., Mathieu, C., & Brisebois, H. (2013). Perception of partner abuse and its impact on marital violence from both spouses. *Scientific Research, 4*(11), 858–863. https://doi.org/10.4236/psych.2013.411123.

Bowman, C. G. (2003). Theories of domestic violence in the African context. *Cornell Law Faculty Publications,* Paper 131. http://scholarship.law.cornell.edu/cgi/viewcontent.cgi?article=1130&context=facpub.

Bradley, S. (2018). Domestic and family violence in post-conflict communities: International Human Rights Law and the state's obligation to protect women and children. *Health and Human Rights Journal, 20*(2), 123–136.

Bragg, H. L. (2003). *Child protection in families experiencing intimate partner violence.* US Department of Health and Human Services, Administration for Children and Families.

Breiding M. J., Chen J., & Black M. C. (2014). *Intimate partner violence in the United States—2010.* National Center for Injury Prevention and Control, Centers for Disease Control and Prevention.

Campbell, J. C. (2002). Health consequences of intimate partner violence. *The Lancet, 359*(9314), 1331–1336.

Department of Justice. (2013, July). Experience of domestic violence: findings from the 2008/09 to 2010/11 Northern Ireland Crime Surveys. Retrieved November 22, 2015, from https://www.dojni.gov.uk/sites/default/files/publications/doj/nics-2008-09-to-2010-11-domestic-violence-bulletin.pdf.

Doyle, J., & McWilliams, M. (2018). Intimate partner violence in conflict and post-conflict societies: Insights and lessons from Northern Ireland. https://pure.ulster.ac.uk/en/publications/intimate-partner-violence-in-conflict-and-post-conflict-societies.

Duchesne, S., & Haegel, F. (2005). *L'entretien collectif* [The collective interview]. Armand Colin.

Ellsberg, M., Jansen, H. A., Heise, L., Watts, C. H., & Garcia-Moreno, C. (2008). Intimate partner violence and women's physical and mental health in the WHO multi-country study on women's health and domestic violence: An observational study. *Lancet, 371*(9619), 1165–1172.

Futures Without Violence. (2012). *The facts on health care and domestic violence*. http://www.futureswithoutviolence.org/userfiles/file/HealthCare/ HealthCare.pdf.

Ganley, A. L., & Schechter, S. (1996). *Intimate partner violence: A national curriculum for children's protective services*. Family Violence Prevention Fund.

García-Moreno, C., Pallitto, C., Devries, K., Stöckl, H., Watts, C., & Abrahams, N. (2013). *Global and regional estimates of violence against women: Prevalence and health effects of intimate partner violence and non-partner sexual violence*. Geneva, Switzerland: World Health Organization. http://apps.who. int/iris/bitstream/10665/85239/1/9789241564625_eng.pdf.

Gupta, J., Reed, E., Kelly, J., Stein, D. J., & Williams, D. R. (2012). Men's exposure to human rights violations and relations with perpetration of intimate partner violence in South Africa. *Journal of Epidemiology and Community Health, 66*(6), https://doi.org/10.1136/jech.2010.112300.

Huecker, M. R., & Smock, W. (2020, January). *Domestic violence* [Updated October 15, 2020]. In StatPearls [Internet]. Treasure Island (FL): StatPearls Publishing. Available from: https://www.ncbi.nlm.nih.gov/books/NBK499 891/.

IGIHE. (2017, February 6). Domestic violence: 64 killed, 10 suicides in 2016. *IGIHE Network*. http://en.igihe.com/news/domestic-violence-64-killed-10-suicides-in-2016.html.

Izugbara, C. O., Obiyan, M. O., Degfie, T. D., & Bhatti, A. (2020). Correlates of intimate partner violence among urban women in sub-Saharan Africa. *PLoS ONE, 15*(3), https://doi.org/10.1371/journal.pone.0230508.

Kayibanda, J. F., Bitera, R., & Alary, M. (2012). Violence toward women, men's sexual risk factors, and HIV infection among women: Findings from a National Household Survey in Rwanda. *Journal of Acquired Immune Deficiency Syndrome, 59*(3), 300–307. https://doi.org/10.1097/QAI.0b013e318 23dc634.

Kelly, J. T. D., Colantuoni, E., Robinson, C., & Decker, M. R. (2018). From the battlefield to the bedroom: a multilevel analysis of the links between political conflict and intimate partner violence in Liberia. *BMJ Global Health, 3*(2), https://doi.org/10.1136/bmjgh-2017-000668.

Kinyanda, E., Weiss, H. A., Mungherera, M., Onyango-Mangen, P., Ngabirano, E., Kajungu, R., Kagugube, J., Muhwezi, W., Muron, J. & Patel, V. (2016). Intimate partner violence as seen in post-conflict eastern Uganda: Prevalence, risk factors and mental health consequences. *BMC International Health and Human Rights, 16*(5), https://doi.org/10.1186/s12914-016-0079-x.

Krug, E. G., Dahlberg, L. L., Mercy, J. A., Zwi, A. B., & Lozano, R. (Eds.). (2002). *World report on violence and health*. World Health Organization. http://whqlibdoc.who.int/publications/2002/9241545615_eng.pdf?ua=1.

L'Écuyer, R. (1989). L'analyse développementale du contenu [The developmental analysis of content]. *Revu de L'Association Pour La Recherche Qualitative, 1*, 51–80.

L'Écuyer, R. (1990). *Méthodologie de l'analyse développementale de contenu: Méthode GPS et concept de soi* [Methodology of the developmental analysis of content: Method of GPS and self-concept]. Presses de l'Université du Québec.

Miles, M. B., & Huberman, A. M. (1994). *Qualitative data analysis: An expanded sourcebook* (2nd ed.). Sage.

Ministry of Gender and Family Promotion [MIGEPROF]. (2011a). *National policy against gender-based violence*. Kigali, Rwanda: Author. http://www.mig eprof.gov.rw/fileadmin/_migrated/content_uploads/GBV_Policy-2_1_.pdf.

Ministry of Gender and Family Promotion [MIGEPROF]. (2011b). *National strategic plan for fighting against gender-based violence 2011–2016*. Kigali, Rwanda: Author. http://www.migeprof.gov.rw/fileadmin/_migrated/content_uploads/GBV_Policy_Strategic_Plan-2.pdf.

Molinié, W. (2016, June 29). Violences conjugales: 122 femmes mortes sous les coups de leur compagnon en 2015 [Domestic violence: 122 women killed by their companion in 2015]. *La Chaîne Info*. http://www.lci.fr/faits-divers/violences-conjugales-122-femmes-mortes-sous-les-coups-de-leur-com pagnon-en-2015-1511813.html.

Mukashema, I., & Sapsford, R. (2013). Marital conflicts in Rwanda: Points of view of Rwandan psycho-socio-medical professionals. *Procedia-Social and Behavioral Sciences, 82*(3), 149–168. https://doi.org/10.1016/j.sbspro.2013. 06.239.

NISR [National Institute of Statistics of Rwanda]. (2020). *Size of the resident population 2019*. http://www.statistics.gov.rw/publication/size-resident-population.

NISR [National Institute of Statistics of Rwanda], Ministry of Health, and ICF International. (2012). *Rwanda demographic and health survey 2010* [Final report]. Calverton, MD. https://dhsprogram.com/pubs/pdf/FR259/FR259. pdf.

Ndushabandi, E. N., Kagaba, M., & Gasafari, W. (2016). *Intra-family conflicts in Rwanda: A constant challenge to sustainable peace in Rwanda*. http://www.irdp.rw/wp-content/uploads/2019/02/intrafamily-con flicts-last-version-2.pdf.

Ntaganira, J., Muula, A., Masaisa, F., Dusabeyezu, F., Siziya, S., & Rudatsikira, E. (2008). Intimate partner violence among pregnant women in Rwanda. *BMC Women's Health, 8,* 17. http://www.biomedcentral.com/1472-6874/8/17.

Nybergh, L., Taft, C., & Krantz, G. (2012). Psychometric properties of the WHO Violence Against Women instrument in a male population-based sample in Sweden. *British Medical Journal Open, 2*(6), https://doi.org/10.1136/bmjopen-2012-002055.

Republic of Rwanda. (2016). Law Nº32/2016 of 28/08/2016 governing persons and family. *Official Gazette nº37 of 12/09/2016.*

Rees, S., Tol, W., Mohsin, M., et al. (2016). A high-risk group of pregnant women with elevated levels of conflict-related trauma, intimate partner violence, symptoms of depression and other forms of mental distress in post-conflict Timor-Leste. *Translational Psychiatry, Nature, 6,* 1–7. https://doi.org/10.1038/tp.2015.212.

Rubanzana, W., Ntaganira, J., Freeman, M. D., & Hedt-Gauthier, B. L. (2015). Risk factors for homicide victimization in post-genocide Rwanda: A population-based case-control study. *BMC Public Health.* http://www.biomedcentral.com/1471-2458/15/809.

Rubin, H. J., & Rubin, I. S. (1995). *Qualitative interviewing: The art of hearing data.* Sage.

Rubin, H. J., & Rubin, I. S. (2005). *Qualitative interviewing: The art of hearing data* (2nd ed.). Sage.

Rutayisire, T., & Richters, A. (2014). Everyday suffering outside prison walls: A legacy of community justice in post-genocide Rwanda. *Social Science and Medicine, 120,* 413–420. https://doi.org/10.1016/j.socscimed.2014.06.009.

Saile, R., Neuner, F., Ertl, V., & Catani, C. (2013). Prevalence and predictors of partner violence against women in the aftermath of war: A survey among couples in northern Uganda. *Social Science and Medicine, 86,* 17–25. https://doi.org/10.1016/j.socscimed.2013.02.046.

Sarabwe, E., Richters, A., & Vysma, M. (2018). Marital conflict in the aftermath of genocide in Rwanda: An explorative study within the context of community based sociotherapy. *Intervention, 16*(1), 14–21.

Schechter, S. (2000). *New challenges for the battered women's movement: Building collaboration and improving public policy* [Online]. https://vawnet.org/sites/default/files/materials/files/2016-09/BCS1_col.pdf.

Shamu, S., Abrahams, N., Temmerman, M., Musekiwa, A., & Zarowsky, C. (2011). A systematic review of African studies on intimate partner violence against pregnant women: prevalence and risk factors. *PLoS ONE, 6*(3), https://doi.org/10.1371/journal.pone.0017591.

Shipway, L. (2004). *Intimate partner violence: A handbook for health professionals*. Routledge.

Thomson, D. R., Bah, A. B., Rubanzana, W. G., & Mutesa, L. (2015). Correlates of intimate partner violence against women during a time of rapid social transition in Rwanda: Analysis of the 2005 and 2010 demographic and health surveys. *BMC Women's Health, 15,* 96. https://doi.org/10.1186/s12905-015-0257-3.

United Nations Office on Drugs and Crime. (2013). The many faces of homicide. In United Nations Office on Drugs and Crime (Ed.), *Global study on homicide 2013: Trends, contexts, data* (pp. 49–57). https://www.unodc.org/documents/gsh/pdfs/Chapter_2-2.pdf.

Umubyeyi, A., Persson, M., Mogren, I., & Krantz, G. (2016). Gender inequality prevents abused women from seeking care despite protection given in gender-based violence legislation: A qualitative study from Rwanda. *PLoS ONE.* https://doi.org/10.1371/journal.pone.0154540.

Umubyeyi, A., Mogren, I., Ntaganira, J., & Krantz, G. (2014). Intimate partner violence and its contribution to mental disorders in men and women in the post-genocide Rwanda: Findings from a population-based study. *BMC Psychiatry, 14,* 315. https://doi.org/10.1186/s12888-014-0315-7.

Verduin, F., Engelhard, E. A. N., Rutayisire, T., Stronks, K., & Scholte, W. F. (2012). Intimate partner violence in Rwanda: The mental health of victims and perpetrators. *Journal of Interpersonal Violence, 28,* 1839–1858. https://doi.org/10.1177/0886260512469106.

Were, E., Curran, K., Delany-Moretlwe, S., Nakku-Joloba, E., Mugo, N. R., Kiarie, J., Bukusi, E. A., Celum, C., & Baeten, J. M. (2011). A prospective study of frequency and correlates of intimate partner violence among African heterosexual HIV serodiscordant couples. *AIDS, 25*(16), 2009–2018. https://doi.org/10.1097/QAD.0b013e32834b005d.

WHO [World Health Organization]. (2012). *Understanding and addressing violence against women: Intimate partner violence*. World Health Organization.

WHO [World Health Organization]. (2013). *Global and regional estimates of violence against women: Prevalence and health effects of intimate partner violence and non-partner sexual violence.* https://apps.who.int/iris/handle/10665/85239.

9

Child- and Youth-Headed Households: An Alternative Solution to Chaotic Family Situations in Post-genocide Rwandan Society

Immaculée Mukashema

Introduction

Estimations from 2005 concluded that 290,000 children younger than eighteen years in Rwanda were orphans, and this was one of the highest numbers worldwide of children who have lost both parents (UNICEF, 2006). In sub-Saharan Africa, the number of double orphans without any relatives is increasing (Barnett, 2005; UNICEF, 2006). East and Southern Africa has been confronted with a growing number of child- and youth-headed households since the 1980s, and this was linked to the impacts of the AIDS epidemic (Ayieko, 1997; Evans, 2005; Foster et al., 1997). The large number of orphans without any adult relatives in Rwanda (Boris et al., 2006; UNICEF, 2007) was due to the combined effects of the 1994 genocide and the HIV/AIDS epidemic (Ntaganira et al., 2012). AIDS orphans exhibited higher levels of mental distress

I. Mukashema (✉)
College of Arts and Social Sciences, University of Rwanda, Butare, Rwanda

than those who were orphaned by genocide or other causes (Caserta et al., 2016).

The dual impact of violent conflict and the HIV/AIDS epidemic has led to dramatic changes in family units and systems of care and created radical shifts in the composition of households (Barnett, 2005; Christiansen, 2005). This trend is seen as a symbol of the social safety net breaking down (Roalkvam, 2005). While the presence of an adult seems to protect children from abuse and facilitate access to resources (Ruiz-Casares, 2009), older siblings are generally the ones in charge of running the household as well as raising income in the settings of what is known as child- and youth-headed households (Ruiz-Casares, 2009).

Estimations state that the genocide has left 10% of children aged 0–18 years old as orphans (Pells, 2012; Thurman et al., 2008). Ten years after the genocide against the Tutsis, UNICEF (2004) estimated that 101,000 people were living in 42,000 YHH (youth-headed households) in Rwanda. UNICEF (2009) has stated that in the 1990s, for example, Rwanda had one of the highest proportions of youth-led families in the world and today, over 100,000 children are believed to live in such households. A study by Mirza (2006) has stated that about 10% (65,000 households) and over 300,000 children were living within youth-headed households in Rwanda; and that among those youth-headed households, 90% were headed by girls, placing young girls at a higher risk of sexual exploitation and transactional sex (Mirza, 2006). Orphans and YHH are particularly vulnerable to maltreatment because of marginalization from the community (Ntaganira et al., 2012).

With the decline in the traditional systems that included long-standing approaches to fostering orphans, a new phenomenon has emerged whereby young people are heading households as a "family" without parents. The phenomenon of leading the households by children or by youths is due to the fact that their parents died due to conflict, genocide, or disease. These child- and youth-headed households are seen by many as signaling a breakdown in social stability (Roalkvam, 2005). The naming of child-headed households (CHHs) or of youth-headed household (YHHs) depends on the definition of child and of youth in countries where the households are headed by orphans and occupied by younger siblings. A CHH phenomenon is defined as a family unit headed by the oldest person who is under the age of 18 (UNICEF, 2010). While the YHH is similar to the CHH, the head of the youth-headed household is older than the child age. In child-headed households and in youth-headed households, the oldest sibling becomes the head of the household and fulfills the responsibility of caring for the younger siblings (Schaal & Elbert, 2006; Van Breda, 2010; Veale et al., 2001). The orphans take on adult roles they had not been prepared for (Ntuli et al., 2020).

Most African orphans have been absorbed into informal fostering systems (Masmas et al., 2004; Monasch & Boerma, 2004). Such systems, however, are increasingly overwhelmed, and many orphans head households (Deininger et al., 2003; Watts et al., 2005). The number of children heading households in sub-Saharan Africa is reported to be growing (Ayieko, 1997). A survey conducted in South Africa in 2006 showed that 122,000 (0.67%) of the country's children were living in child-headed households (Meintjes et al., 2009).

While the number of orphans in many countries of sub-Saharan Africa is increasing on the one hand, on the other hand, there is a move from community-oriented living towards a greater individualization of social organization (see, for example, Hertrich & Lesclinigand, 2001). In Rwanda this move is occurring despite the country's strong emphasis on community and consensual approaches to problem solving. Indeed, the traditional family and extended family structures suffered a grave blow as a consequence of the genocide against the Tutsi and its aftermath (MIGEPROF, 2011).

Youth-headed households are still a relatively new phenomenon about which little is known (Evans, 2010; Uwera et al., 2012). However, it is clear that these households share some principal characteristics: They form a "family" that provides support and continuity (McAdam-Crisp, 2006); they deal with the adult responsibilities of supporting themselves at an age when the care and the protection of an adult are normally needed (Schaal & Elbert, 2006); and they assume an anthropological and psychosocial position for which they were never prepared (Boris et al., 2006).

However, it is as yet unclear how these youth-headed households deal with conflict in the households. Since researches show that conflict is a part of family life where adults are generally present in that conflict occurs between husband and wife, between parent and child (e.g., Canary & Canary, 2013; Malek, 2010), and between siblings (e.g., Canary & Canary, 2013; Furman & Buhrmester, 1985; Howe et al., 2002; Malek, 2010)—this begs the question: How do children acting as the head of a family of siblings deal with the inevitable family conflict? Not only are these family units made up of siblings, but they are also siblings living in a new form of alternative family (see Bartoszuk & Pittman, 2010), caring for younger siblings and fulfilling other adult responsibilities in the absence of adult supervision. Further, when there is conflict between siblings living in traditional families, parents can intervene; but in a youth-headed household the siblings are obliged to live together, as siblings and as "special" family members, in a lifestyle and pattern of authority initiated by their parents but continued in a non-traditional structure that has been arrived at with no choice in the matter. Spouses in traditional families choose freely to get married and live together, while the youth-headed household does not involve choice by all parties. The head of a youth-headed household lacks the moral authority that accompanies public support of the parental role: "you should obey your parents," but no one says you should obey your brother or your sister.

The research described here investigated conflict and dissension between siblings living in youth-headed households as a new kind of "alternative family" (Bartoszuk & Pittman, 2010). The research sought to answer the following questions:

1. What are the characteristics of the youth-headed households that participated in the present study?
2. Do members of such households believe that there is undue conflict and dissension in their youth-headed households?
3. What do household members perceive to be the causes of conflict or dissension?
4. What are the consequences of these conflicts?
5. How do youth-headed household members feel when conflict or dissension occurs?

6. What strategies do youth-headed household members use to deal with conflict and dissension? What can be done to help these families headed by young people to achieve a healthy life?

Methods

Field, Population of the Study, and Selection of Participants

This research was conducted in Huye District, in its four administrative sectors: Ngoma, Mbazi, Gishamvu, and Rwaniro. Huye is one of the Districts of the Southern Province in Rwanda. In Huye District, the population is estimated at 319,000 and, as in other Districts of Rwanda, that population is young, with 52% aged 19 or younger (NISR, 2012a). In Huye District, 3% of the population aged 0–20 years is composed of double orphans, the national rate being 2.7% (NISR, 2012a).

A qualitative method based on the "basic interpretative research" approach (Merriam, 2002) was selected. This approach is recommended for research when little is known on the topic to be explored (Grenier, 2005), such as the nature of conflict and dissension management among the members of a household headed by a youthful sibling examined in the present research. We gathered our data in focus group discussions because these interactions are known to help capture youth experiences more effectively than structured survey research (see, for example, Berg, 1995). Further, over time it has been shown that focus group discussion generates data that is extremely rich and of high quality (Ashar & Lane, 1991), and that this method has a unique ability to generate data based on the synergy and the stimulation of the group interaction (Catterall & Maclaran, 1997; Hess, 1968) because group members influence each other by responding to ideas and comments in the discussion (Krueger & Casey, 2000).

Seven focus group discussions were conducted. These groups were composed of double orphans who were heading households of siblings and who agreed freely and voluntarily to give information about conflict and dissension in their homes. Selection and recruitment of participants was facilitated by the local administration in collaboration with two non-governmental organizations called, respectively, "Association Modest et Innocent (AMI)" and "*Igiti cy'Ubugingo Centre (IUC)*". These two NGOs work with double orphans living in youth-headed households in the four administrative sectors, which were in a rural area. The data collection was carried out between December 2011 and January 2012 at convenient locations in the four administrative sectors.

Research Approach

Two moderators including the principal investigator and two assistants were recruited from among our colleagues on the basis that they had experiences with the community and were therefore comfortable in engaging the youth participants. The moderators underwent two days of training on how to conduct focus group discussions and on the ethics of research with human being as participants. The moderators were provided with a guiding agenda of research questions in Kinyarwanda, the national local language, to use as the tool for the discussions. Keeping in mind the overall research objective of seeking to understand conflict and dissension between siblings living in youth-headed households, the research guide was constructed so that participants could answer open-ended questions pertaining to each to the following themes:

1. the participants' beliefs about the existence of undue conflict and dissension in their youth-headed households;
2. the perceptions of the participants as household members with respect to the causes of such conflict or dissension;
3. the consequences of conflict and dissension on the households;
4. the feelings of youth-headed household members when conflict or dissension occurs;
5. the strategies used by youth-headed household members to deal with conflict and dissension; and
6. recommendations from the participants on what can be done to assist these families achieve a healthy life.

Additionally, in order to generate further information, the moderators asked probing questions during the interview sessions to assist with the clarification of ideas. Each participant signed an informed consent form, and an authorization permitting the recording of the discussion was obtained at the start of each focus group session. With one exception where only female participants were available, separate and parallel sessions were conducted for each gender, to maximize the homogeneity of group members (Brown, 1999) and thus facilitate easy communication. The total number of focus group discussions was seven and included four to seven participants. To promote a relaxed environment during the sessions, participants were given a soft drink as refreshment. At the end of each session participants were financially compensated by receiving 1500 Rwandan francs (RWFs) or about $2 US for the day spent traveling to the location of the session and the time spent in the focus group discussion.

Data Analysis

The method of data analysis was based on the approach to content analysis developed by L'Écuyer (1989, 1990). This method shows the essential stages of content analysis by identifying themes and subthemes in what is expressed by participants on a given topic. All seven tapes from the seven focus group discussions were transcribed into seven transcripts, producing a total of ninety-four pages. These were translated from Kinyarwanda into English. The Kinyarwanda and English versions were then read repeatedly by the principal investigator to "absorb the content" of the discussions (Baribeau, 2009).

The narratives contained in the transcripts were analyzed in order to locate the points of view given by the participants in response to the questions posed in connection with the objective of the study (Duchesne & Haegel, 2005). The coding was carried out using NVIVO as software for qualitative data coding, which helped in the elaboration of the codes (Duchesne & Haegel, 2005). Every line, paragraph, and/or section of text was given a specific code. As the coding progressed, the code definitions continued to be challenged and new codes were developed when properties were identified in the data that did not fit the existing codes. During the data analysis, there was constant movement between the raw data and the analysis (see Baribeau, 2009; Glaser & Strauss, 1967; L'Écuyer, 1989; Paillé, 1994) and constant comparison of categories and codes in each new transcript. The purpose was to fully develop overarching categories for each individual group code. The process was continued until no new code emerged.

Results and Discussion

Data of this qualitative and exploratory research are presented under the following broad headings relating to the semi-structured interview guide previously described: characteristics of the participants; the existence and signs of conflict and dissension in youth-headed households; the causes of conflict in youth-headed households; consequences which arise from conflict and dissension; the feelings of the heads of households when conflict and dissension occur; means used by youth-headed households to cope with conflict and dissension; the expressed needs of youth-headed households for coping with conflict; and measures that could be taken to help the youth-headed households mitigate the effects of serious conflict and dissension.

Characteristics and Structure of the Focus Group Discussion

Table 9.1 summarizes some basic information about the groups. See Column D for the total number of participants. In Column F, the acronym YHH stands for "youth-headed household."

Column A shows the number identifying the focus groups discussions from 1 to 7. The first focus group is identified as 11, the second as 21, the third as 31, the fourth as 41, the fifth as 51, the sixth as 61, and the seventh focus group is identified as 71. Column B pertains to the gender of the participants and shows that focus groups 11, 41, and 71 are composed of male participants, while focus groups 21, 31, 51, and 61

Table 9.1 Characteristics and structure of the focus group discussions (FGDs)

A	B	C	D	E	F	G
Identi-fying # of the FGD[a]	Gender of the members of FGD[a]	Ages and age range of the participants in FGD[a]	Number of FGD members[a]	Smallest and largest size of households headed by the participants in the FGDs[a]	Period headed/lived in the current YHHs (years)[a]	Range of monthly income estimations in RWFs ($1USD = approx. 650 RWFs) < means less than[a]
1	Male	19; 20; 21; 24; 26; 17 (range: 17–26)	6	2–5	12; 4; 8; 4; 3; 4	<10,000; <0,000; <10,000; <10,000; <10,000; <10,000
2	Female	28; 31; 22; 23; 17; 23; 21 (range: 17–31)	7	2–8	18; 17; 2; 2; 2; 4; 5	<10,000; <10,000; <10,000; <10,000; <10,000
3	Female	24; 21; 21; 29; 24; one missing (range: 21–29)	6	2–4	2; 5; 4; 4; 3	Range 10,000–30,000; <10,000; <10,000; <10,000
4	Male	17; 20; 21; 21 (range: 17–21)	4	2–3	3; 4; 1; 17	Range 10,000–30,000; Range 10,000–30,000; Range 10,000–30,000; Range 10,000–30,000
5	Female	24; 20; 20; 17; 23; 17 (range: 17–24)	6	2–5	2; 9; 9; 1; 6; 1	<10,000; <10,000; <10,000; <10,000
6	Female	19; 30; 20; 20; 21; 18 (range: 18–30)	6	2–7	1; 17; 9; 3; 4; 4	Range 10,000–30,000; Range 10,000–30,000; <10,000; <10,000; Range 10,000–30,000; <10,000
7	Male	25; 28; 24; 22; 22; 27 (range: 22–28)	6	2–5	17; 15; 13; 4; 17; 6	<10,000; <10,000; <10,000; <10,000
			Total: 41			

[a]Explanation of the information contained in Table 9.1

are composed of female participants. Column C lists the ages of all the participants in the study and the age range of each of the focus groups. Participants who were 21 years of age at the time of the data collection constitute the largest single age group (7 out of a total of 41 participants), followed by participants aged 20 (6 out of 41), and those aged 17 and 24 (each age contributing 5 participants out of 41). Column D shows that the size of the focus groups varied from 4 to 7 participants.

For each household headed by the participants in focus group discussions, Column E indicates the smallest and the largest number of household members. For example, the smallest size among the households headed by the participants in focus group discussion 11 is 2 people, while the largest household comprises 5 people. Similarly, the smallest number of members among the households headed by the participants in focus group discussion 21 is 2 while the largest is 8. Looking at the sizes of the households headed by the participants in general in Column E, the households ranged from 2 members to a high of 8 members. These household sizes limits are similar to the general size of households in Rwanda where 84% of households have between two and seven members (NISR, 2012b).

Column F shows respectively the period that the participants have been heading or living in the youth-headed households. The time spent without parents is ranged from 1 to 18 years. The presentation of the ages in Column C and the duration of time in Column F are done respectively. This means, for example, that the first participant in focus group 11 is aged 19 years (first in Column C) and has been living in his youth-headed household for 12 years (first in Column F). The next participant in focus group 11, who is aged 20 years (second in Column C), has been living in his youth-headed household during 4 years (same participant as second in Column F).

There are two observations here: Some participants lived in youth-headed households before they actually became the head of the household, for example, when the head left the family in order to marry. For this reason, in Table 9.1, some participants have the same age or almost the same age as the time they have spent in the current youth-headed household. One 21-year-old participant—the third participant in the Columns C and F for focus group 11—said that he had been living in his youth-headed household for 8 years. Otherwise, this participant should have been heading his household at the age of 21 years minus 8 years, or at 13 years of age, which was not the case. However, there were also many participants who were less than 18 when their parents died and they had started to act as head of households. This accords with previous observations (see, for example, Thurman et al., 2006; Ward & Eyber, 2009).

Column G shows the monthly income of each participant as they mentioned it at the time of the data collection. The presentation of the mentioned monthly income is made in the same respective order as in Columns C and F. Even though there are difficulties with the concept of income in predominantly agricultural countries, and people living on subsistence agriculture may not be good at computing the value of their produce, the majority of participants said they have a household income of less than 10,000 Rwandan francs per month (less than $15 US per month); this means that participants are extremely poor. The average consumption per poor adult equivalent in real terms in 2011 was RWFs 123,891 at the national level (NISR, 2012b) and RWFs 106,754 in the Southern Province (NISR, 2012a). At the national level, 44.9% of the population are identified as poor, and 56.5% in the Southern Province (NISR, 2012a), where Huye District is located. The National Institute of Statistics report (NISR, 2012a, 2012b) does not clearly state if the average consumption reported is per year or per month. Still, overall, there is no doubt, based on the data, that the majority of youth-headed household members are very poor.

Existence and Signs of Conflict and Dissension in Youth-Headed Households

As was expected, conflict and dissension does exist in youth-headed households and tends to manifest in reclusiveness and a lack of positive interaction between members of the household. The experience can be summed up in the following example:

[Y]ou prefer loneliness or directly you go to bed, whereas you should share the meal prepared by your brother who remained at home...we can spend all the night brawling; they are quarrelling unceasingly, it is always the brawl between them. (11)

Causes of Conflict in Youth-Headed Households

Drinking, the use of drugs, harassing others, young female family members becoming pregnant, the selfishness of the oldest (and some of the other household members), property and disagreement around the sharing of property (and income): These are said to be the causes of conflict in households headed by young people. Participants expressed the sources of conflict by saying:

As far as I am concerned, I have got an unintended child, I have my little sister and she does not respect me and she always tells me that I have given birth to an illegal child and this always causes conflict. (21)

When these children take or use drugs, they enter into perpetual/everlasting conflict and this may even lead them to kill each other. (41)

Conflict among non-accompanied children may result from the fact that there is no one to teach them to behave, as for most of the time you see them in the same age range. (71)

You may live for example with your young brothers and sisters and take care of them, but little by little when you become old enough and mature you become selfish and forget to look after them. (21).

As my friends mentioned, when children live alone, sometimes the eldest becomes impossible and feels that he/she can't get advice from his/her younger brothers/sisters, and thus acts like a dictator towards them. (61)

A major source of conflict reported across groups is a lack of agreement on issues related to property left by the parents, such as such the land and the cows—disagreement on the sharing out of property that was held in common in the youth-headed households. These disagreements were described as follows:

The dissensions can come from the possessions that your parents left you. If you are the elder one of the family, you may be guided by your own interests to the detriment of your brother. You can for example sell a field [land] without informing your brother. When he finds out, he will complain, wanting to know why you did it without him knowing. Thus, conflict may occur between you, because what you do, you do without consulting him, since your heritage is common and shared. (31)

When one of the members gets married, it is also said to be a time of conflict/dissension.

There were some cows at home and my elder brother got married and then he wanted to take them to his household and we refused and this created conflict among us. (71)

Siblings in youth-headed households are victims of poverty and hunger that make it difficult for them to get on well. The households are not able to satisfy the basic needs of their members and that situation may lead them into conflict and dissension. As the participants noted:

Poverty problems may result in conflict...It happens that you lack something to eat and conflict may occur from this situation. (21)

In concrete terms, it has been said that conflict often results from poverty, which prevent children in the family from getting on well with each other. Indeed, you can find children who have no parents but live together in harmony because they are never in need. So, you can't realize that they are orphans because they don't come into conflict, thanks to their well-being. (51)

In terms of the sharing of responsibility, youth-headed household members think that it is not only the head (who has to be playing the parental role) who is responsible for getting household needs met; each sibling member of the household who is able to do so needs to make a contribution. As one of the participants said:

> For example, if they want to grow beans, they ask the eldest to buy the seed, but he/she has no means; so, when he/she suggests that everybody should contribute, they disagree with him/her and insist that it's up to the eldest to provide the seed. And thus the conflict starts. (51)

In the youth-headed households as well as in other kind of families, the failure to take and fulfill responsibilities is a source of discord and dissension.

Consequences that Arise from Conflict and Dissension in Youth-Headed Households

Consequences of dissension in youth-headed households, as in other families, may include members leaving home and the break-up of the family. Examples to illustrate these points are related by participants in the following examples:

> When there is conflict, a child can flee the family and go in the street to become a "street child." (11)

> The first consequence is to leave the family home and to go to wander in the street. (41)

> They can leave the house, each going his own way, and live a vagabond life. (61)

When there is conflict or dissension, some sibling members of youth-headed households do not try to deal with it but leave the home. Leaving home may be aimed at searching for better living conditions, but this may end in failure. This failure can be translated, for a girl, in the experience of an unwanted pregnancy:

If it is a girl, she may not go in the street but she may unintentionally fall pregnant because you do not get along suitably in your family...you may find, for example, some child who fails to live in the family and prefers to live and go to town and when she gets pregnant there she comes back and finds you there without any sufficient means to take care of her. (11)

The consequence of conflict/dissension in youth-headed households may be mental suffering and drug abuse, as in these examples:

You will understand that he/she has a mental disease like trauma, etc. (71)

Now, I have stomach pains. Very recently, I had a stomach attack...you may feel your heart subjugated by sadness...You may miss the sleep; you may have a generalized malaise, etc. (31)

Drug abuse as a refuge may lead to or itself constitute health problems expressed in mental suffering and in physical illness:

If there are problems in the family, they take refuge in the consumption of drugs and other narcotics. (31)

You may start taking drugs in order to soothe the pain and forget many things you meet in life. (71)

Besides, his/her younger brothers suffer from it enormously. (11)

In situations of conflict and dissension in youth-headed households, if members are not fully capable of work this lead to poverty:

From this situation, the families' members cease to work, become poor, and then conflicts increase...Because of living in disagreement and misunderstanding, you do not work, and you become poor. (21)

Another consequence may be extreme poverty because when there is conflict you cannot work in order to develop yourselves...A severe consequence, as I told you, from my experience, is poverty. (71).

There is the poverty which is due to the misunderstandings in general. (11)

The consequence I find is that they never achieve what they had planned, because of those conflicts. (51)

Feelings of Heads of Households When Conflict and Dissension Is Present in Their Families

The heads of household who participated in this research reported a variety of feelings and emotions. These are related to psychological distress, to social isolation from neighbors and from the support of the authorities, to neighbors who made the conflict between siblings worse, to lack of motivation, and to suicidal thoughts and negative sentiments about themselves as heads of household. One example follows:

[It] is the feeling of loneliness and lack of motivation to do something because you do not see any good coming from doing something…lack of people who show they care for you by talking to you, to such an extent that you feel you are hating all people…If you have a problem you lack a neighbor who can come and comfort you…When conflicts occur, frankly speaking, my experience is that no one cares about these orphan children. (71)

Living in conflict and dissension make the heads of households feel stressed, discouraged, and abandoned by a society that does not care about them. Some report feeling like abnormal people. Others remarked on an absence of anyone they could approach for comfort, be it neighbors or authorities. They reported that when they needed to talk to an authority figure, they were afraid to approach that person. They feel abandoned and socially isolated. In turn, because of this feeling of social isolation, they prefer to keep quiet and not tell anyone about their conflict-related problems:

There are moments when one is really in distress, moments when there is nobody who approaches you to comfort you and even the authorities do not come to see you; you never see them...you feel lost. Even when you would need to talk to an authority, you are afraid to approach it...we live in extreme conflict...I did not understand, I even wanted to commit suicide...Sometimes, one decides to commit suicide. (31)

Participants reported that in cases of conflict and dissension in their family, the neighbors do not help to solve conflict but instead say things to the elder or younger brother of the head that are intended to worsen the situation and even harm the children's property:

As children living alone, we often face several problems. Neighbors despise us, and harm our property because we don't have any support-...With this, neighbors themselves make life difficult for you, because you don't have any friend among them who can take your defense...-Sometimes you find yourself in a bad neighborhood, but you can't do anything about it. You are aware that you live only thanks to God's will, and not others' will. (61)

This is consistent with the assertion that some neighbors act spitefully toward the young heads of households. Youth-headed households feel a lack of motivation to deal with their responsibilities. They have no motivation to work and may fall into depression, realizing that their previous actions are ineffective:

The consequence is the feeling of loneliness and lack of motivation to do something because you do not see any good coming from doing something...lack of people who care for you by talking to you to such an extent that you feel you are hating all people. (71)

Sometimes sibling members of youth-headed households living in discordant circumstances have suicidal thoughts. This may be due to conflict, but also may also be linked to situations of social isolation, negative emotionality, and depressive symptoms. Some household members may decide to move far away from their siblings when there is conflict and dissension in their families. The unhealthy situation can lead the heads of youth-headed households to regret being the eldest of the family, as they fear to approach the authorities to speak about their problems:

Most of the time we first lose self-control and regret being the eldest in the family, because of the problems. So, we feel swamped by events but manage to support them, since there is no other solution; sometimes you ask yourself why you are still alive, and you wish you had died. (51)

The feelings of this YHH are consistent with those of double orphans who are heading households in Uganda who experienced their situation as a huge and complex problem for themselves as well as for people in their villages. However, these situations could improve if actions focused on practical and psychological issues as well as on sensitization about the children's situation could be initiated. In addition to the fact that these children need adult guidance to become citizens who act in accordance with the expectations in their communities, material aid is important in order to reduce the children's experiences of being "different" and constantly experiencing survival anxieties (Dalen et al., 2009).

Means or Strategies Employed by Youth-Headed Households to Face up to Family Conflict

In order to cope with conflict and dissension, participants reported sharing their concerns with peers and people of the same age enduring the same experience, their own friends or a parent's friends. Members of youth-headed households reported that they mainly prefer to talk to people with the same experience of conflict and dissension, preferably other young people, their peers, when discussing their experiences and seeking help in finding solutions, rather than having recourse to older people:

Instead of making recourse to the old people…better is that young people of your age intervene in your problems (a girl or a boy), contrary to what adults can do…Another means is to invite another young person of your age to come to intervene in your problems in order to help you to reconcile. (11)

It is necessary to seek people who have the same problems as you to talk about it. One exposes his; the other does the same thing. After that, each one feels relieved; each one feels calm and less worried in his heart. (31)

When heads of sibling households encounter family discord, they can go to their own friends or the friends of their dead parents and ask them to intervene with their advice. In conflict and dissension situations, they would be willing to search for help in the extended family—an aunt or uncle—but in general such family members no longer exist:

I run to contact other family members like my aunt because the neighbors do nothing but telling my elder or younger brother things that are intended to worsen the situation...You try among the family members even though you sometimes lack them. You may lack an aunt or uncle. (71)

Needs in Relation to Conflict and Dissension Between Siblings in the Youth-Headed Households

Youth-headed households reported on what they think can be done in order to assist sibling-headed families to no longer exist in serious situations of conflict and dissension. They were clear that what they need most of all is economic assistance and psychosocial support:

Financial help for poverty reduction is helpful, because most of the time conflicts come from poverty. (21)

I think that there should be organizations which can deal with the studies of these children since they are intelligent. Those who cannot reach secondary studies can profit from vocational training which will help them to fend for themselves in their future like the others. (31)

For my part, I need assistance so that I can get my own home, because I'm about to be chased from where I'm living now...We need your help because, as the eldest of the family, we are like parents for our young brothers and sisters. When they need something you are unable to find, such as lotion, soap or food, you are overtaken by problems. I think you should help us. (51)

Clearly, the participants in this study need economic assistance to be helped out of poverty. Youth-headed households need to be approached by counselors and advisers and they need advocacy. Heads of household said that they needed advice, counseling, advocacy, and adult guidance:

In these problems especially lies the conflict that is found in children-led households...their lack of willingness to solve those problems because these children do not have anyone to advocate for them...frankly speaking, my experience is that no one cares about these orphan children. Orphans, as they lack means, should have people who advocate for them in law, in the courts, because there are many people who have problems in courts and lack advocacy because they do not know the laws and are victimized in front of the law. (71)

Youth-headed households need to be approached regularly and specifically by community leaders, neighbors, and friends. This can help them, especially those who are very young, to overcome the lack of role models, as they put it. It would also help them to deal with the feeling of being marginalized within community structures and give them guidance. As they noted:

Sometimes, children-headed families lack proper education...Beside this, when one takes drugs, this worsens the situation and makes you live in disagreement or conflict. (41)

Conflict among children without parents may result from the fact that there is no one to help them in how to behave, as for most of the time you are with people in the same age range. You notice that some of them drink beer or take drugs whereas other do not, which is seen as a problem which has the potential to separate them or generate misunderstanding among them. (71)

Actions to Be Taken

There is an urgent need for siblings in youth-headed households to be specifically approached in a helpful and supportive way by leaders, counselors, and advisers. There is also an urgent need for advocacy:

> I find that it is good that there is an adviser with whom to exchange ideas; but a mature person, who is capable, not a child as we are, so that we can develop. (11)

> To have counselors and advisers for everyday life...There should be people who can train and advise children-headed families about their everyday life and show them how they can handle their problems when they occur...Neighbors, friends, people to be near them and advise them to live in peace. (21)

> We also need advocacy. (71)

Youth-headed households also need the community leaders to approach them in order to help them in solving their problems:

> Leaders should approach orphans to know their problems in order to solve them properly...There should be a meeting of children who live together where they discuss their problems. Even one meeting in three months may be sufficient. (21)

> They [the authorities] should set up a secure place where they can find these children...One wonders how he will live; when you do not have somebody, an authority to listen to you, to look into your problems, you feel lost. Thus we would like them to approach us where we are, in our villages, our cells, and our sectors...strongly encourage all the basic authorities to take care of the survival of these children, to know how they live from day to day. (31)

> They should schedule a day when we can meet and discuss our problems. This is how they can be informed about the problems each child has...I have never seen any intervention of the authorities when it comes to

children to live alone or care for other children. When we are called in general you do not have ways to give your ideas. If you are an authority who cannot take at least one day a year to visit those children, you cannot know their problems. What I am telling you is true…You cannot know what the child thinks or that there are people who want to harm him in different ways if you don't talk to him. (71)

Mentoring interventions cost little, and have been shown to be effective in a variety of settings (Dubois et al., 2002). Successful mentoring programs may also help to renew social interconnectedness in Rwanda (Boris et al., 2006). Specific structures may need to be put in place to deal with the issues of daily life and regulation confronting youth-headed households. The findings of this study suggest that it is very important to pass laws that specifically recognize the existence of youth-headed households and regulate and support their rights and duties in the same way as the laws that govern other kinds of families. These laws should also deal with the property of such households.

In a country that has a high number of youth-headed households (Lee, 2012) that is likely to increase because traditional foster care is declining, such special measures are clearly necessary. As the older members of these households take over the parental role at an early age and in an unusual way, following the death of their parents, they face challenges that sometimes cause them to regret their seniority in the family. Specific strategies should be put in place to support them in order to preserve their mental health. One such strategy would be to set up a specific and clear structure for their material and psychosocial support.

Because so many members of the youth-headed households that participated in this study stated that they feel a lack of motivation to action, a sense of isolation, and a lack of administrative and social support, this research suggests that it is important to set up a specific national structure to employ strategies dealing with all of the daily life issues experienced in such households. Included in these policies and approaches should be a special channel of effective advocacy for youth-headed households. Our data shows that there is currently no specific institution that supports youth-headed households; they have nowhere to go where they can find advocacy specific to their needs.

This chapter focuses on the resilience of children facing extreme hardship and adversity. It is based on participatory research with children living in child-headed households in Rwanda. It emphasizes the importance of listening to children's voices and recognizing their capacities when designing interventions to strengthen their psychosocial well-being. This study shows that children have developed innovative and profitable coping strategies and some have even developed the capacity to thrive through their situation of extreme hardship. The study of these coping strategies suggests that the children displayed resourcefulness, responsibility, and a sense of morality. However, when the stressors in a child's life became too great, they tended to employ negative, and potentially harmful, strategies to cope. A community-based approach should focus on strengthening overall community well-being, and should aim to build on the capacities of children, such as their positive coping mechanisms and resilient characteristics. At the same time, it should appropriately address their areas of vulnerability. Existing protective factors should also be identified and further developed in interventions (Ward & Eyber, 2009).

These youth-headed households constitute a new kind of alternative family with a unique structure and social and demographical characteristics that need official recognition and the rights associated with that recognition. These youth-headed households require specific regulations that give them the same rights that are enjoyed by traditional adult-headed households. These rights would enable siblings in youth-headed families to have the same entitlement to socio-economic support—(e.g., the V2020 *Umurenge* program, one of the strategic programs for fighting poverty in Rwanda)—as adult-headed families, and thus to emerge from the poverty that is one of the causes of conflict and dissension. Further, youth-headed households should be provided with training in family responsibilities, responsibilities like parenting and family management. As one focus group participant explained:

Counselors can also help these children by teaching and training them. The government has a role to play as well...we want people who can come closer to us and advise us. (71)

The main aspects—signs, causes, and consequences—of conflict and dissension are present even in traditional families and in other types of alternative families (Malek, 2010; Mukashema & Sapsford, 2013; Slegh & Kimonoyo, 2010). The youth-headed households in general and those living in conflict and dissension are unique, however, in that no adult member of any other family can say that he or she needs "adult support" to solve family problems. This means that youth-headed households are constantly aware of their vulnerabilities and lack of resources. On the other hand, they have demonstrated their capacity to cope with life events and, through that, their resilience in the face of the most unfavorable situation that of being orphans without an adult presence in their family lives.

Conclusion

This chapter discussed youth-headed households (YHHs) in post-genocide Rwanda. It informed about the signs of conflict and dissension in youth-headed households, its causes, its consequences, and the feelings of the heads of these households when conflict and dissension are present. The chapter also described the means used to face these situations, the needs of the household heads in relation to such conflict and dissension between siblings, and their expressed needs so that they can be helped to no longer live with such serious discord.

Conflict does exist in youth-headed households. The most common post-conflict responses of family members are withdrawal and lack of positive interaction between members of the household. Dissension and conflict are most often triggered by behaviors such as drinking, the use of drugs, harassing others, engaging in sexual activity that leads to unintended pregnancy, the perceived selfishness of the oldest (and some other household members), different views about property and property-sharing, and disagreement around the property (and income) sharing. Additionally, siblings in youth-headed households are often the victims of poverty and hunger that compound the difficulty in getting on well with each other. These young people are unable to satisfy the basic needs of their household members and so these privations and conditions of daily life almost inevitably lead to conflict and dissension. The consequences of conflict and dissension in youth-headed households, as in other families, are that family members leave home, endure mental suffering and drug abuse, and that some families completely break apart. Likewise, if members are not fully capable of work, the family suffers from poverty, underlining and reinforcing the cycle of conflict in the family.

The young people who live in youth-headed households where there is conflict and dissension experience psychological distress, social isolation from neighbors, lack of support from authorities, disengagement from neighbors who often make the conflict between siblings worse, and they also show lack of motivation, suicidal thoughts, and negative sentiments about themselves as heads of household. Young heads of households often lack motivation to deal with their responsibilities. In order to face conflict and dissension, participants reported sharing their experience with peers and people of the same age and same experience, including their own friends or a parent's friends.

Implications

This chapter showed that youth-headed households are distressed households whose members need economic assistance and psychosocial support. These households require outreach from counselors and advisers and they need advocacy and guidance. It is therefore recommended that specific structures be put in place to deal with all issues in their daily life for regulation. Judging by the research outputs presented in this research chapter, it seems to be of the utmost importance for the Rwandan Government to write legislation that recognizes the existence of youth-headed households (YHHs) and enshrines their rights and responsibilities in the same way as is done with the existing laws governing other kinds of families. Mental health and psychosocial interventions should be designed to reduce psychological distress among youth-headed households' members.

Not all child-headed households (CHHs) and youth-headed households (YHHs) are made of orphans today in Rwanda. From observation and from various media reports in Rwanda, there is an emerging phenomenon of adolescent pregnancy that leads to child-headed households (CHHs) and youth-headed households (YHHs). The vulnerable girl, the child-mother, whose rights are violated, may be obliged to create her own household to live in with her child and this happens in obviously inappropriate normal living conditions. Yet adolescent pregnancies are a global problem and 777,000 girls under 15 years give birth each year in developing regions around the world (UNFPA, 2015; UNICEF, 2013; WHO, 2020). A research is necessary (1) to understand the psychosocial and economic living conditions of that category of female children and adolescents; (2) to make updates on estimations of child and youth-headed households in post-genocide Rwanda.

Acknowledgements I am very grateful to the former National University of Rwanda (NUR) in general, to the former NUR's Research Commission and Sida Sarec in particular, for the financing of this research. Many thanks also to Professor Roger Sapsford for his assistance.

An early version of this chapter was presented to the third Asian conference on psychology and behavioral sciences, March 28–31, 2013, Osaka, Japan; and published as "The challenging absence of adults in youth-headed households: the case of dissension management among the family members of households headed by a sibling in Rwanda" in the *International Journal of Child, Youth and Family Studies*, 5(2.1): 354–374. https://doi.org/10.18357/ijcyfs.MukashemaI.5212014. A new analysis including the data's aspects of child- and youth-headed households in post-conflict Rwandan society as well as the implications from the findings was conducted.

References

Ashar, H., & Lane, M. (1991). Focus groups: An effective tool for continuing higher education. *Journal of Continuing Higher Education, 41*(3), 9–13. https://doi.org/10.1080/07377366.1993.10400881.

Ayieko, M. (1997). From single parents to child-headed households: The case of children orphaned by AIDS in Kisumu and Siaya districts—Study paper (No. 7). United Nations Development Program (UNDP).

Baribeau, C. (2009). Analyse des entretiens de groupe [Analysis of group interviews]. *Recherches Qualitatives, 28*(1), 133–148.

Barnett, T. (2005). HIV/AIDS, childhood and governance: Sundering the bonds of human society. *African Journal of AIDS Research, 4*(3), 139–145. https://doi.org/10.2989/16085900509490353.

Bartoszuk, K., & Pittman, J. F. (2010). Does family structure matter? A domain specific examination of identity exploration and commitment. *Youth and Society, 42*(2), 155–173. https://doi.org/10.1177/0044118X10377648.

Berg, B. (1995). *Qualitative research methods for social sciences* (2nd ed.). Allyn and Bacon.

Boris, N. W., Thurman, T. R., Snider, L., Spencer, E., & Brown, L. (2006). Infants and young children living in youth-headed households in Rwanda: Implication of emerging data. *Infant Mental Health Journal, 27*(6), 584–602. https://doi.org/10.1002/imhj.20116.

Brown, J. B. (1999). The use of focus groups in clinical research. In B. F. Crabtree & W. L. Miller (eds.), *Doing qualitative research* (2nd ed., pp. 109–124). Sage.

Canary, H. E., & Canary, D. J. (2013). *Family conflict: Managing the unexpected*. Polity.

Caserta, T. A., Pirttilä-Backman, A. M., & Punamäki, R.-L. (2016). Stigma, marginalization and psychosocial well-being of orphans in Rwanda: Exploring the mediation role of social support. *AIDS Care, 28*(6), 736–744. https://doi.org/10.1080/09540121.2016.1147012.

Catterall, M., & Maclaran, P. (1997). Focus group data and qualitative analysis. *Sociological Research Online, 2*(1). http://www.socresonline.org.uk/2/1/6.html.

Christiansen, C. (2005). Positioning children and institutions of childcare in contemporary Uganda. *African Journal of AIDS Research, 4*(3), 173–182. https://doi.org/10.2989/16085900509490356.

Dalen, N., Nakitende, A. J., & Musisi, S. (2009). "They don't care what happens to us." The situation of double orphans heading households in Rakai District, Uganda. *BMC Public Health, 9*(321). https://doi.org/10.1186/1471-2458-9-321.

Deininger, K., Garcia, M., & Subbarao, K. (2003). AIDS-induced orphanhood as a systemic shock: magnitude, impact and program interventions in Africa. *World Development, 31*(7), 1201–1220. https://doi.org/10.1016/S0305-750X(03)00061-5.

Dubois, D. L., Holloway, B. E., Valentine, J. C., & Cooper, H. (2002). Effectiveness of mentoring programs for youth: A meta-analytic review. *American Journal of Community Psychology, 30*(2), 157–197. https://doi.org/10.1023/A:1014628810714.

Duchesne, S., & Haegel, F. (2005). *L'entretien collectif* [The collective interview]. Armand Colin.

Evans, R. (2005). Social networks, migration and care in Tanzania: Caregivers' and children's resilience in coping with HIV/AIDS. *Journal of Children and Poverty, 11*(2), 111–129. https://doi.org/10.1080/10796120500195527.

Evans, R. (2010). *The experiences and priorities of young people who care for their siblings in Tanzania and Uganda (Technical Report).* Reading, UK: University of Reading, School of Human and Environmental Sciences, Department of Geography and Environmental Sciences. https://pdfs.semanticscholar.org/0d61/ae49e64ca752966e1bfd844d50b8d38745ab.pdf.

Foster, G., Makufa, C., Drew, R., & Kralovec, E. (1997). Factors leading to the establishment of childheaded households: The case of Zimbabwe. *Health Transition Review, 7,* 155–168. http://www.jstor.org/stable/40652332.

Furman, W., & Buhrmester, D. (1985). Children's perceptions of the qualities of sibling relationships. *Child Development, 56*(2), 448–461. https://doi.org/10.2307/1129733.

Glaser, B. G., & Strauss, A. L. (1967). *The discovery of grounded theory: Strategies for qualitative research.* Aldine Publishing Co.

Grenier, S. (2005). Paradoxe et opportunité de la recherche qualitative en santé mentale communautaire [Paradox and opportunity of qualitative research in community mental health]. Recherches qualitatives-Hors-Série-Numéro 1. *Actes de colloques Recherche Qualitative et production des savoirs.* UQAM, 12 mai 2004. http://www.stes-apes.med.ulg.ac.be/Documents_electroniques/MET/MET-DON/ELE%t20MET-DON%20A-8136.pdf.

Hertrich, V., & Lesclinigand, M. (2001). *Transition to adulthood in rural Africa: Are male and female experiences converging? The case of the Bwa of Mali.* XXXIV Congrès Général de la population, Salvador, Brazil, August 18–24, 2011. Paris: INRD.

Hess, J. M. (1968). Group interviewing. In R. L. King (Ed.), *New science planning* (pp. 51–84). American Marketing Association.

Howe, N., Rinaldi, C. M., Jennings, M., & Petrakos, H. (2002). No! The lambs can stay out because they got cozies: Constructive and destructive sibling conflict, pretend play, and social understanding. *Child Development, 73*(5), 1460–1473. https://doi.org/10.1111/1467-8624.00483.

Krueger, R., & Casey, M. (2000). *Focus groups: A practical guide for applied research* (3rd ed.). Sage.

L'Écuyer, R. (1989). L'analyse développementale du contenu [The developmental analysis of content]. *Revu de L'Association Pour La Recherche Qualitaitive, 1,* 51–80.

L'Écuyer, R. (1990). *Méthodologie de l'analyse développementale de contenu: méthode GPS et concept de soi* [Methodology of the developmental analysis of content: Method of GPS and self-concept]. Presses de l'Université du Québec.

Lee, L. (2012). *Strategies to support youth-headed households in Kenya and Rwanda* (Backgrounder Number 43). Centre for International Governance Innovation.

Malek, C. (2010). *Family conflict.* University of Colorado.

Masmas, T. N., Jensen, H., Da Silva, D., Høj, L., Sandström, A., & Aaby, P. (2004). The social situation of motherless children in rural and urban areas of Guinea-Bissau. *Social Science and Medicine, 59*(6), 1231–1239. https://doi.org/10.1016/j.socscimed.2003.12.012.

McAdam-Crisp, J. L. (2006). Factors that enhance and limit resilience for children of war. *Childhood, 13*(4), 459–477. https://doi.org/10.1177/090756 8206068558.

Meintjes, H., Hall, K., Marera, D.-H., & Boulle, A. (2009). *South Africa's youngest parents.* SA News. South African Government News Agency.

Merriam, S. B. (2002). *Qualitative research in practice: Examples for discussion and analysis.* Jossey-Bass.

Mirza, S. (2006). Childhood bypassed: Rwanda's youth-headed households. *SAIS Review of International Affairs, 26*(2), 179–180. https://doi.org/10.1353/sais.2006.0039.

MIGEPROF [Ministry of Gender and Family Promotion]. (2011). *Strategic plan for the integrated child rights policy in Rwanda.* Kigali: Government of Rwanda. http://ncc.gov.rw/IMG/pdf/ICRP_Strat_Plan_FINAL_290911. pdf.

Monasch, R., & Boerma, J. T. (2004). Orphanhood and childcare patterns in sub-Saharan Africa: An analysis of national surveys from 40 countries. *AIDS, 18,* S55–S65. https://doi.org/10.1097/00002030-200406002-00007.

Mukashema, I., & Sapsford, R. (2013). Marital conflict in Rwanda: Points of view of Rwandan psycho-socio-medical professionals. *Procedia-Social and Behavioral Sciences, 82*(2013), 149–168. https://doi.org/10.1016/j.sbspro. 2013.06.239.

NISR [National Institute of Statistics of Rwanda]. (2012a). The third Integrated Household Living Conditions Survey (EICV3): District profile–South–Huye. Kigali. http://www.statistics.gov.rw/publication/eicv-3-huye-district-profile.

NISR [National Institute of Statistics of Rwanda]. (2012b). The third Integrated Household Living Conditions Survey (EICV3): Main indicators report. Kigali. https://www.statistics.gov.rw/publication/eicv-3-main-indicators-report.

Ntaganira, J., Brown, L., & Mock, N. B. (2012). Maltreatment of youth heads of households in Rwanda. *Rwanda Journal of Health Sciences, 1*(1). https://www.ajol.info/index.php/rjhs/article/view/82341.

Ntuli, B., Sebola, E., & Madiba, S. (2020). Responding to maternal loss: A phenomenological study of older orphans in youth-headed households in impoverished areas of South Africa. *Healthcare, 8*(3), 259. https://doi.org/10.3390/healthcare8030259.

Paillé, P. (1994). L'analyse par théorisation ancrée [The analysis by anchored theorization]. *Cahier de Recherche Sociologique, 23*, 147–181. https://doi.org/10.7202/1002253ar.

Pells, K. (2012). "Rights are everything we don't have": Clashing conceptions of vulnerability and agency in the daily lives of Rwandan children and youth. *Children's Geographies, 10*(4), 427–440. https://doi.org/10.1080/14733285.2012.726072.

Roalkvam, S. (2005). The children left to stand alone. *African Journal of AIDS Research, 4*(3), 211–218. https://doi.org/10.2989/16085900509490360.

Ruiz-Casares, M. (2009). Between adversity and agency: Child and youth-headed households in Namibia. *Vulnerable Children and Youth Studies, 4*(3), 238–248. https://doi.org/10.1080/17450120902730188.

Schaal, S., & Elbert, T. (2006). Ten years after the genocide: Trauma confrontation and post-traumatic stress in Rwandan adolescents. *Journal of Traumatic Stress, 19*(1), 95–105. https://doi.org/10.1002/jts.20104.

Slegh, H., & Kimonoyo, A. (2010). *Masculinity and gender-based violence in Rwanda: Experiences and perceptions of men and women.* Rwanda Men's Resource Centre.

Thurman, T. R., Snider, L. A., Boris, N. W., Kalisa, E., Nyirazinyoye, L., & Brown, L. (2008). Barriers to the community support of orphans and vulnerable youth in Rwanda. *Social Science & Medicine, 66*(7), 1557–1567. https://doi.org/10.1016/j.socscimed.2007.12.001.

Thurman, T., Snider, L., Boris, N., Kalisa, E., Mugarira, E., Ntaganira, J., & Brown, L. (2006). Psychosocial support and marginalization of youth-headed households in Rwanda. *AIDS Care: Psychological and Socio-medical Aspects of AIDS/HIV, 18*(3), 220–229. https://doi.org/10.1080/09540120500456656.

UNFPA [United Nations Population Fund]. (2015). *Girlhood, not motherhood: Preventing adolescent pregnancy*. New York.

UNICEF [United Nations Children's Fund]. (2004). *Rwanda: Ten years after the genocide*. http://www.unicef.org/infobycountry/rwanda_genocide.html.

UNICEF [United Nations Children's Fund]. (2006). *Africa's orphaned and vulnerable generations: Children affected by AIDS*. http://www.unicef.org/publications/files/Africas_Orphaned_and_Vulnerable_Generations_Children_Affected_by_AIDS.pdf.

UNICEF [United Nations Children's Fund]. (2007). *Une aide pour les orphelins du Rwanda* [Help for the orphans of Rwanda]. http://assets.unicef.ch/downloads/fsheet_ruanda_050725_fr_neu.pdf.

UNICEF [United Nations Children's Fund]. (2009). *UNICEF Rwanda Background*. Retrieved from http://www.unicef.org/infobycountry/rwanda_1717.html.

UNICEF [United Nations Children's Fund]. (2010). *Children and AIDS: Fifth Stocktaking Report, 2010*. United Nations.

UNICEF [United Nations Children's Fund]. (2013). *Ending child marriage: Progress and prospects*. UNICEF.

Uwera, K. C., Brackelaire, J. L., & Munyandamutsa, N. (2012). La fratrie dans les ménages d'enfants sans parents au Rwanda après le génocide [Siblingship in households without parents in Rwanda after the genocide]. *Dialogue, 2*(196), 61–72. https://doi.org/10.3917/dia.196.0061.

Van Breda, A. D. (2010). The phenomenon and concerns of child-headed households in Africa. *Sozialarbeit Des Südens, 3*, 259–279.

Veale, A., Quigley, P., Ndibeshye, T., & Nyirimihigo, C. (2001). *Struggling to survive: Orphans and community dependent children in Rwanda*. Report for Ministry of Local Government and Social Affairs, UNICEF, Trócaire, and Care International. Dublin: Trócaire. https://www.unicef.org/evaldatabase/index_15410.html.

Ward, L. M., & Eyber, C. (2009). Resilience of children in child-headed household in Rwanda: Implication for community-based psychosocial interventions. *Intervention, 7*(1), 17–33. https://doi.org/10.1097/WTF.0b013e32832ad3ac.

Watts, H., Lopman, B., Nyamukapa, C., & Gregson, S. (2005). Rising incidence and prevalence of orphanhood in Manicaland, Zimbabwe, 1998 to 2003. *AIDS, 19*(7), 717–725. https://doi.org/10.1097/01.aids.0000166095.62187.df.

WHO (2020, January 31). *Adolescent pregnancy*. https://www.who.int/news-room/fact-sheets/detail/adolescent-pregnancy.

10

General Conclusion

Immaculée Mukashema

Introduction

Rwandan society and probably all human communities within middle-
and low-income countries need professional marriage and family therapy,
but the contextualization of approaches to psychosocial and cultural
values of those communities is essential. There is a view of culturally
sensitive framework for interventions that is based on the concept of
conceptualism, which emphasizes that an individual must be understood
within the context of his or her family, and that at the same time, the
family needs to be understood within the context of the culture in which
it is immersed (Bernal, 2006; Bernal & Sáez-Santiago, 2006).

However, in the context of Rwandan society and probably in the
context of societies with similarities, it is hard to find existing literature
on marriage and family life therein. The similarities of those societies can
be based on the facts that they are: (1) middle- and low-income countries'

I. Mukashema (✉)
College of Arts and Social Sciences, University of Rwanda, Butare, Rwanda

I. Mukashema (ed.), *Psychosocial Well-Being and Mental Health of Individuals
in Marital and in Family Relationships in Pre- and Post-Genocide Rwanda,*
https://doi.org/10.1007/978-3-030-74560-8_10

societies, (2) post-conflict societies. Lack of literature on marriage and family life becomes more complicated when it relates to ancient times of those societies, and the connection between the past and the current times. This volume is about sharing researches' outputs emerging from within and inside pre- and post-genocide Rwanda, through exploratory qualitative research approaches. This volume is an attempt to fill the gap in existing literature on marriage and family life, and to serve as a milestone in the progress of public health towards better well-being of the spouses and family members and thus of the society made by families at large.

Components of the Book

Our book intends to contribute to evidencing that psychosocial interventions aimed at marriage and family well-being should take into account the past and present socio-cultural context the beneficiaries of psychosocial interventions are in. It is important to remember that the family is the smallest traditional social cell/unit of the overall world society, but that each society has its own uniqueness with the general common characteristics within the whole world. That uniqueness cannot be left behind in programming for the marriage and family well-being in the society.

This book would bring in a more contextual mindset to the implementation and the evaluation of interventions in mental health and well-being in the post-genocide Rwandan society by drawing on its past positive culture. While being evidence-based, the book also aims to contribute to influencing policymakers and individual practitioners in the area of marriage and family in terms of how interventions are designed and implemented.

The book is composed of ten chapters including an introductory chapter and the present conclusion chapter. Chapter 1 presents and shows in details the reasons that have led to the title of the whole book "Psychosocial Well-Being and Mental Health of Individuals in Marital and in Family Relationships in Pre- and Post-Genocide Rwanda."

Chapter 2 is about the qualitative research approaches used in exploring marriage and family life in ancient Rwandan society. The chapter introduces the overall research project on psychosocial well-being and mental health in marriage and family within Rwandan pre-genocide society. It gives details on the research methods applied to the research findings presented and discussed in Chapters 3–7.

Chapter 3 gives an overview of the characteristics of marital life in traditional Rwandan society. It shows that marital life in pre-genocide Rwandan society was characterized by societal pressure and spousal awareness about compliance with cultural values in marital life. The societal pressure and spousal awareness about compliance with cultural values in marital life were key to building strong households in Rwanda society. Normal marital life functioning traditionally was arranged that spouses would see each other as equal, as different, and as complementary human beings. Those perspectives about how spouses saw each other brought harmony to their marital lives. In addition, and equally important, was the fact that the marital lifestyle in ancient Rwandan society was a good way of preparing children for marriage. The parents in the traditional Rwandan society would play a fundamental role in the whole marriage process of their children.

Chapter 4 is about the determinants of marital happiness as a dimension of marital quality in ancient Rwandan society. Healthy marriage and marital happiness were related to the achievement of the reasons why people would get married. Abiding by cultural conditions of good marital functioning was key to healthy marriage and a happy marital life in ancient Rwandan society. The reasons why people got married and subsequently enjoyed marital happiness included having children, getting an increased social support through the ties established with the other family, and experiencing an increase of their own wealth. The conditions of happiness which were related to the spousal marital life functioning included respect toward the in-law family members, collaboration of both spouses in contributing to the increase of wealth of the household, good communication between spouses, common marital life direction, mutual respect coupled with obeying each other, love and balanced power relations among the spouses, and ultimately the living of marital life in a peaceful manner.

Chapter 5 is about the socio-cultural causes of marriage destruction in the ancient Rwandan society. Marital conflict is obvious in each marriage and the ancient Rwandan society did not make an exception to this reality. However, divorce resulting from marital conflict was not seen as an option to solve marital problems in ancient Rwandan society. There were efficient family and cultural mechanisms used to deal with the spousal disputes within the families without leading to divorce. Specific cases could lead to divorce and were culturally accepted. These were cases of adultery, the discovering of a hidden disease or/and malformation in one of the spouses after marriage, marital sexual relation dissatisfaction, dirtiness and lack of hygiene, drunkenness, disrespect, stealing, and infertility. Bad behaviors like adultery were common to both wives and husbands. Some behaviors like dirtiness and disrespect were specifically considered for women, while bad behaviors like stealing (especially family resources in the context of this study) and the like could be particularly seen in men.

The situation of marital conflict was not alarming in ancient Rwanda. The attempt to explain the non-alarming marital conflict in ancient Rwandan society is two-fold. First, there were cultural values that would prevent the spouses from making marital conflicts publicly known. Second, marital conflict in new homes of ancient Rwandan society was prevented through young age upbringing in their family of origin. New spouses would behave the way they had observed over the marital life course of their parents. These latter would bear in mind and do all they could so that their behavioral action in front of their children could not have a negative impact on them—especially on their future marital life.

Chapter 6 is about protective factors of marriage lastingness in the traditional Rwandan society. Spouses' families of origin had an important place and consideration in the new spouses' marital life and functioning in ancient Rwandan society. This place and consideration was an important factor in marriage lastingness in ancient Rwandan society. New spouses had a psychosocial responsibility of preventing anything that could break the family ties established between their two respective families of origin. The spouses had an exceptional commitment to marital life functionality. Spouses were able to show patience and mutual respect to each other as well as perseverance in their marital life.

Chapter 7 explores and reports on the ways which were used to deal with destructive marital conflict in customary Rwanda. Normal and good marital lifestyle of the parents was a good practical way of teaching the children about marital life. The children would learn by observation of how marital life functions. Learning by observing their parents' marital lifestyle would help their children in their future marriages, and thus prevent destructive marital conflict in the new households made up by the children. In addition, destructive marital conflict was prevented through verbal pieces of advice given to the young lady and the young boy just prior to their marriage.

Whenever conflict arose despite the prevention processes, destructive marital conflict was first managed within the new household by the spouses themselves. In case of need, the two families would help the spouses to resolve the conflict. These two families of origin were crucial in the new destructive spousal marital conflict management and resolution once the conflict was not solved by the spouses by themselves. While helping the spouses in destructive conflict, the families would abide by the principle of objectivity. Spouses could make recourse to the "Kwahukana" phenomenon, a situation in which a spouse (generally the wife) could sometimes flee the marital home for a relatively short period, in a situation of destructive marital conflict. She would flee to her family-in-law or to her family of origin. Following this separation, the management of the conflict could be carried out in the family where the wife had fled. Both families were supportive to the new spouses in cases of marital conflict to such an extent that the family-in-law of the married woman could even protect and defend her.

From where the woman had taken sanctuary and sometimes in the presence of the two families together, the husband would only succeed in getting her wife back home after he had discussions on the reasons that had caused the spousal conflict in question. Deliberations were always fair and would end in blaming the wrongdoer in the conflict. The spouses, especially the wives, were reminded about the need for having patience and perseverance in marital life. The husband, more specifically, was warned about the wrong done and the need for him to be a good head of the household. Four main reasons were behind the efforts of the new spouses and the two families of origin in preventing and eventually in dealing fairly with marital conflict in ancient Rwandan society: (1) building a stable and well functioning new household, (2), preventing divorce, (3) making the new household last long, and (4) maintaining the ties established between the two families of origin.

Chapter 8 reports on intimate partner violence in post-genocide Rwandan society. The data were collected in three districts of Southern Province and Western Province of Rwanda, using qualitative research approaches. Results revealed that women easily report economic abuse and physical violence but needed support from other people to report sexual violence, and generally did not report psychological harassment, perhaps because they accepted it as a social norm. Men generally did not report intimate partner violence (IPV) and the main victims of IPV in all its forms were children and women. A number of measures can help to reduce IPV. These include among others: economically empowering females; educating and sensitizing family members about their responsibilities and community leaders about laws and human rights; educating all community members about gender equality and IPV including premarital instruction; increasing access to services; putting in place a law that protects free unions by giving them legal status after a period of cohabitation; setting up a specific institution to deal with IPV; improving both support to the victims and follow-up of reported cases, along with instituting punitive responses to deter potential new perpetrators.

Chapter 9 is about looking at conflict and dissensions in new types of alternative families of post-genocide Rwandan society. These particular alternative families are composed of siblings, and headed by one of the siblings. They are known as children- and youth-headed households. The chapter arises from an exploratory study in which qualitative data was collected. Seven focus group discussions were conducted with the heads of forty-one youth-headed households in post-genocide Rwanda. Like in other types of families, conflict and dissension are common in youth-headed households. Conflict and dissensions are manifested in poor communication and absence of positive interaction between members. The most often reported consequences of this conflict and dissension include household members leaving home and becoming separated from the family, and this is coupled with and exacerbated by health problems and poverty.

Participants also reported feeling psychological distress, social isolation, lack of motivation, and suicidal thoughts. Where there is conflict, participants turn to their own friends or their parents' friends for support. Participants also reported needing economic assistance and psychosocial support. Based on the focus group interviews, the researcher concludes that it would be beneficial to set up specific community-based structures that can deal with all the issues of daily life and regulation facing youth-headed households. The researcher recommends that the training of youth-headed households in how to take on family responsibilities should be a national policy. This chapter forms a conclusion to the book.

Main Insights from the Book

The findings from various researches and presented in the book show that ancient Rwandan marital and family members had specific ways and behaviors in their marriage and family relations that were based on its cultural and societal contexts. From the findings about the overview of the characteristics of marital life as they are presented in Chapter 3; the determinants of marital happiness as dimension of marital quality as presented in Chapter 4; the socio-cultural causes of marriage destruction presented in Chapter 5; the protective factors of marriage lastingness presented in Chapter 6; up to the findings about the ways which were used to deal with destructive marital conflict in customary Rwanda as are presented in Chapter 7, we can say that the whole research illustrates and supports Ndushabandi et al. (2016) statement that raises the awareness on the necessity of avoiding contradictions between legal provisions and Rwandan traditional gender practices and Rwanda's culture while dealing with family and of course marriage issues.

Fitting of the Book's Content in the Sustainable Development Goal 3 (or SDG 3) and Applicability in Other Contexts Similar to Rwanda

The family is an important environment of the psychosocial life of its members. The family well-being can ensure the well-being of its members. This volume fits the Sustainable Development Goal 3 (or SDG 3) as one of the seventeen sustainable development goals established by the United Nations in 2015. The SDG 3 is about good health and well-being and aims to ensure healthy lives and to promote well-being for all at all ages across all races (United Nations, 2015).

The link between SDG 3 and the current book is that the aim and the vision of both go hand-in-hand. This is the achievement of mental health and well-being for the spouses and family members in Rwanda in particular, and in all societies similar to Rwanda. Once the spouses and family member are healthy and have well-being within their societies, the SDG 3 target will be achieved. As researchers who contributed to this book, we make an academic contribution to inform policymakers about mental psychosocial support policies aligning the cultural values.

This book supports Thomas et al. (2017) idea suggesting that it is important for health promotion policies to take into account, among other aspects, the complexities in family relationships, paying attention to family context and relationship quality to benefit health and well-being. The importance of this book is also that it stresses Broderick and Schrader (1991), Jithoo and Bakker (2011), as well as Sholevar's (2003) statements that historical family counseling has emerged from research and practice based on the Western context and thus, there is a need for taking into account the uniqueness of the interactions families have with major environmental systems, in applying the Western models to the African and other similar contexts (Jithoo & Bakker, 2011).

Limitations of the Book and Directions for Further Researches

The book is about an exploratory view of "Psychosocial Well-Being and Mental Health of Individuals in Marital and in Family Relationships in Pre- and Post-Genocide Rwanda." The discussions about the findings presented in Chapters 3–7 are made mainly in relation to existing literature. However, even if the literature used fits in terms of the domains of the academic works, not all the literature fits the cultural and societal contexts of the findings from Rwandan participants. Nevertheless, the explanation of this limitation is that this book is among the first, if not the only one to date, in the area of marriage and family life and well-being in pre- and post-genocide Rwandan society. There are no previous academic publications on marital and family well-being in Rwanda, or on intimate violence and the phenomenon of children and youth-headed household in pre-genocide Rwandan society. Another limitation concerns the samples of the research participants in the various studies presented in this book. These participants were selected and recruited, and the qualitative data were collected and analyzed, via appropriate scientific research approaches; but none of the studies presented were designed to be conducted throughout the whole Rwandan country. However, it is to recall that the country is small geographically of 26,338 km², and that its population shares globally a same culture and a same native language.

Conclusion

Despite some limitations shown above, this volume stands as a milestone for guidance in the evolutionary cultural perspective of marital and family well-being in Rwandan society, and in other similar societies having their specific cultural contexts, and affected by war and genocide. Further researches would benefit in being conducted with the aim of extending marriage and family research to the whole of Rwandan society; to conceptualize and theorize marriage and family well-being in Rwandan society; to investigate the factors and skills influencing the increase in marital satisfaction after marriage; to study intimate partner violence in pre-genocide Rwandan society; to study the phenomenon of alternative families including child- and youth-headed households in pre-genocide Rwandan society; and to elaborate on need for assessment of Rwandans' need of mental health and psychological support. As suggested earlier, further researches are suggested for which customs and values can be taken from the ancient cultures in various societies which have similarities with Rwanda, to make for better and sustainable present-day marriages and family well-being.

References

Bernal, G. (2006). Intervention development and cultural adaptation research with diverse families. *Family Process, 45*(2), 143–151. https://doi.org/10.1111/j.1545-5300.2006.00087.x.

Bernal, G., & Sáez-Santiago, E. (2006). Culturally centered psychosocial interventions. *Journal of Community Psychology, 34*(2), 121–132. https://doi.org/10.1002/jcop.20096.

Broderick, C. B., & Schrader, S. S. (1991). The history of professional marriage and family therapy. In A. S. Gurman & D. P. Kniskern (eds.), *Handbook of family therapy* (Vol. 2, pp. 3–40). Brunner/Mazel.

Jithoo, V., & Bakker, T. (2011). Family therapy within the African context. In E. Mpofu (Ed.), *Counseling people of African ancestry* (pp. 142–154). Cambridge University Press. https://doi.org/10.1017/cbo9780511977350.012.

Ndushabandi, E. N., Kagaba, M., & Gasafari, W. (2016). *Intra-family conflicts in Rwanda: A constant challenge to sustainable peace in Rwanda.* http://www.irdp.rw/wp-content/uploads/2019/02/intrafamily-conflicts-last-version-2.pdf.

Sholevar, G. P. (2003). Family theory and therapy. In G. P. Sholevar & L. D. Schwoeri (Eds.), *Textbook of family and couples therapy: Clinical applications.* American Psychiatric Publishing Inc.

Thomas, P., Liu, H., & Umberson, D. (2017). Family relationships and well-being. *Innovation in Aging, 1*(3), 1–11. https://doi.org/10.1093/geroni/igx025.

United Nations. (2015). *Resolution adopted by the General Assembly on September 25, 2015.* Transforming our world: The 2030 Agenda for Sustainable Development (A/RES/70/1). https://www.un.org/en/develo pment/desa/population/migration/generalassembly/docs/globalcompact/ A_RES_70_1_E.pdf.

Index

The manufacturer's authorised representative in the EU is Springer
Nature Customer Service Centre GmbH, Europaplatz 3, 69115 Heidelberg,
Germany. If you have any concerns regarding our products, please
contact ProductSafety@springernature.com

Printed and bound by CPI Group (UK) Ltd, Croydon, CR0 4YY
29/04/2026
02099478-0004